PERIOPERATIVE NURSING HANDBOOK

PERIOPERATIVE NURSING HANDBOOK

MARK L. PHIPPEN, RN, MN, CNOR

Manager, OR/PACU
The Methodist Hospital
Houston, Texas

MARYANN PAPANIER WELLS, RN, MS, CNOR

Perioperative Nurse Manager, Perioperative Nursing
Hospital of the University of Pennsylvania
Philadelphia, Pennsylvania

W.B. SAUNDERS COMPANY

A Division of Harcourt Brace & Company

PHILADELPHIA   LONDON   TORONTO   MONTREAL   SYDNEY   TOKYO

W.B. SAUNDERS COMPANY

A Division of
Harcourt Brace & Company

The Curtis Center
Independence Square West
Philadelphia, PA 19106

Library of Congress Cataloging-in-Publication Data

Phippen, Mark L.
    Perioperative nursing handbook / Mark L. Phippen, Maryann Papanier
Wells.
        p.   cm.
    ISBN 0-7216-3412-5
    1. Surgical nursing—Handbooks, manuals, etc.   2. Operating room
nursing—Handbooks, manuals, etc.   I. Wells, Maryann M. Papanier.
II. Title.
    [DNLM: 1. Operating Room Nursing—handbooks.   WY 39 P5729p 1995]
RD99.24.P48   1995
610.73'677—dc20
DNLM/DLC   94-25433

PERIOPERATIVE NURSING HANDBOOK   ISBN 0-7216-3412-5

Printed in the United States of America

Last digit is the print number: 9   8   7   6   5   4   3   2   1

PREFACE

The *Perioperative Nursing Handbook* is a user-friendly manual for perioperative nurses and registered nurse first assistants (RNFA). The handbook presents valuable information that the practitioner can use in all phases of the perioperative continuum.

Section I addresses perioperative patient assessment. Use this section as a guide in your assessment activities. Extensive information is provided. In the future, more surgeries will be performed on an outpatient basis, and more patients will be admitted the same day of surgery. Because of this, nurses practicing in outpatient and same day admission units will find that they have a key role in collecting health status data. In fact, the day is coming when the perioperative nurse and RNFA will be the only nurses the patient will see during their surgical and invasive experiences. Assessment skills will become critical for the perioperative nurse of the future.

Section II presents patient outcome standards specific to the perioperative period. Use these standards to develop outcome indicators for quality assessment and improvement activities. Health care of the future will be judged on outcomes.

The practitioner will find Section III useful in the formulation of nursing diagnoses specific to the perioperative period. As we enter a new era in health care, perioperative nurses and RNFAs will be called on to defend their practices and demonstrate their contribution to patient outcomes. Defining perioperative nursing diagnoses will be the first step to demonstrating the perioperative practitioner's contribution to patient outcomes. Use these diagnoses in everyday practice. Take steps to validate the identified risk factors through research.

Sections IV and V present critical competencies for the perioperative nurse and the RNFA. These sections provide guidelines for developing and implementing perioperative nursing and RNFA practice guidelines, perioperative nursing policies and procedures, process and structure indicators for quality assessment and improvement activities, and framework for the development of competency-based perioperative nursing and RNFA performance descriptions and competency-based curricula.

The handbook is compact. Slip it in your pocket and then practice your profession, perioperative nursing.

MARK L. PHIPPEN
MARYANN PAPANIER WELLS

CONTENTS

PERIOPERATIVE PATIENT ASSESSMENT

The purpose of the perioperative patient assessment is to collect sufficient data to enable the perioperative nurse or the registered nurse first assistant (RNFA) to diagnose actual or potential alterations in health patterns that may affect the patient during the perioperative period.

KEY TERMS
Functional Health Patterns

- Provide a framework for identifying potential or actual patient problems. This framework includes assessment of cultural, developmental, and disease phenomena.
- Ensure a holistic assessment, regardless of a patient's age, level of care, or medical disease (Gordon, 1987b).
- Defined as a sequence of health behaviors that occur over time. Functional health patterns are the strengths in a patient's lifestyle (Gordon, 1987b).

Dysfunctional Health Patterns

- Health care problems resolved by nursing activities and known as nursing diagnoses (Gordon, 1987b).
- During the assessment, the patient describes past and present changes in health patterns. The nurse uses this information to identify potential or actual problems that could occur during the perioperative period. Once health problems are identified, the nursing diagnosis can be formulated.

Health Perception–Health Management Pattern

- Describes the patient's "perceived pattern of health and well-being and how health is managed" (Gordon, 1987a, p. 10).
- Provides insight into the patient's ability and desire to adhere to surgical and nursing prescriptions and to participate in the rehabilitation process.

1

- Used to identify the patient's risk for injury, infection, and non-compliance.

Nutritional-Metabolic Pattern

- Describes the patient's pattern "of food and fluid consumption relative to metabolic need and pattern indicators of local nutrient supply" (Gordon, 1987a, p. 11).
- Provides information about the patient's tissue repair process, heat-regulating mechanism, and fluid volume.
- Used to identify the patient's risk for alteration in body temperature, hyperthermia, and hypothermia, impaired skin integrity, fluid volume deficit, and fluid volume excess.

Elimination Pattern

- Describes the patient's "patterns of excretory function (bowel, bladder and skin)" (Gordon, 1987a, p. 11).
- Provides information about the patient's elimination pattern to plan for alterations in bowel, bladder, and skin excretions related to surgical intervention.
- Used to identify the patient's risk for altered postoperative bowel function.

Activity-Exercise Pattern

- Describes the patient's "pattern of exercise, activity, leisure, and recreation" (Gordon, 1987a, p. 11).
- Provides information about the patient's ability to tolerate and recover from the stressors of surgery.
- Used to identify the patient's risk for ineffective breathing pattern, acute pulmonary embolus, ineffective airway clearance, altered tissue perfusion, decreased cardiac output, alteration in postoperative cardiac rate (tachycardia), and self-care deficit following surgery.

Sleep-Rest Pattern

- Describes the patient's "patterns of sleep, rest, and relaxation" (Gordon, 1987a, p. 12).
- Provides information about the patient's ability to engage in restful sleep during the rehabilitation process.
- Used to identify actual or potential sleep-pattern disturbances during the perioperative period.

Cognitive-Perceptual Pattern

- Describes the patient's pattern of auditory, visual, kinesthetic, gustatory, tactile, and olfactory senses, as well as cognitive abili-

ties such as language, memory, and decision making (Gordon, 1987a, p. 12).
- Provides information about the patient's ability to understand instructions and teaching objectives related to the surgical experience.
- Used to identify the patient's knowledge deficit and risk for alteration in comfort.

Self-Perception–Self-Concept Pattern

- Describes the patient's attitudes about body image, identity, sense of worth, emotional pattern, and cognitive and psychomotor abilities (Gordon, 1987a, p. 12).
- Provides information about the patient's ability to deal with psychological stressors such as fear, anxiety, the inability to control a situation, and the disruption of body image and personal identity.
- Used to identify patient fear, anticipatory anxiety, and risk for body image disturbance and self-esteem disturbance.

Role-Relationship Pattern

- Describes the patient's "role engagements and relationships."
- Provides information on how surgery will affect the patient's "perception of the major roles and responsibilities" in his or her current life situation (Gordon, 1987a, p. 12).
- Used to identify the patient's anticipatory grieving.

Sexuality-Reproduction Pattern

- Describes the patient's "satisfaction or dissatisfaction with sexuality" as well as the reproductive pattern.
- Provides information on how surgery will affect the patient's "perceived satisfaction or disturbances in" sexuality and reproductive stage (Gordon, 1987a, p. 13).
- Used to identify the patient's risk for alterations in the sexuality and reproductive pattern.

Coping–Stress Tolerance Pattern

- Describes the patient's "general coping pattern and effectiveness of the pattern in terms of stress tolerance."
- Provides information on how surgery will affect the patient's ability to "resist challenge to self-integrity, modes of handling stress, family or other support systems, and perceived ability to control and manage situation" (Gordon, 1987a, p. 13).
- Used to identify ineffective individual (patient) coping and ineffective family coping.

Value-Belief Pattern

- Describes the patient's "patterns of values, goals, or beliefs . . . that guide choices or decisions."
- Provides information on how surgery will affect the patient's perceptions of what "is important in life and any perceived conflicts in values, beliefs, or expectations" caused by surgery (Gordon, 1987a, p. 13).
- Used to identify actual or potential alterations in the patient's philosophical values and religious beliefs.

Nursing Diagnosis

An actual or potential health problem that is resolved through nursing intervention.

Defining Characteristics

A cluster of signs and symptoms.

Related Factors

The cause of or reason for the health problem.

Risk Factors

Risk factors are elements within the patient's environment that increase the patient's susceptibility to acquire a health problem. The words "high risk for" are used when defining potential health problems (e.g., *high risk for infection*) (Gordon, 1987b).

PERIOPERATIVE PATIENT ASSESSMENT

Currently, the extent of perioperative patient assessment activities will vary according to perioperative nurse/RNFA practice patterns and institutional policies and procedures. In the future, however, with the implementation of health care reform policies and innovations, perioperative nurses and RNFAs will find that their role as health data collectors will expand. They will take a more active role in collecting health data and consequently will become primary identifiers of health problems.

PHYSIOLOGIC ASSESSMENT

The perioperative nurse/RNFA physiologically assesses the patient by

- Collecting baseline vital data
- Obtaining the surgical or invasive procedure history

- Reviewing laboratory and diagnostic studies
- Assessing for allergies and hypersensitivity reactions
- Assessing the integumentary, cardiovascular, respiratory, gastrointestinal, musculoskeletal, and urinary systems.

Collecting Baseline Vital Data

- Take vital signs: pulse, temperature, blood pressure, and respirations.
- Look for abnormal findings (Table 1).
- Communicate abnormal vital signs to the surgeon and the anesthetist.
- Weigh the patient and obtain the patient's height. If measurements are recorded in pounds and inches, also note the metric equivalents.
- Record the patient's chronologic age. If the patient is less than 2 years of age, record the age in months.

Obtaining the Surgical or Invasive Procedure History

- Ask the patient about prior hospitalizations. Obtain the dates and the reason for the hospitalization. If available, include old medical records in the chart.
- Ask about prior surgical and invasive procedures. Obtain the dates of the past procedures and have the patient explain why the procedures were done.
- Ask the patient to describe the outcome of past procedures.
- If the patient had a surgical or invasive procedure in the past, ask about the type of anesthesia that was used and whether there was a reaction to the anesthetic.

Reviewing Laboratory and Diagnostic Studies

Determine what laboratory and diagnostic studies the physician wants ordered, ensure that they are ordered, and ascertain that the results are on the chart. Results of studies should be reviewed to determine whether they are within normal ranges (Tables 2 to 4). If abnormal findings are reported, notify the surgeon and the anesthetist.

- White blood cell count (WBC)
- Red blood cell count (RBC)
- Fasting blood glucose (FBG)
- Urinalysis (UA)
- Blood urea nitrogen (BUN) and creatinine
- Chest radiography
- Electrocardiogram (ECG)
- Other studies (radiologic studies such as angiography and cholangiography, intravenous pyelography, myelography, com-

TABLE 1

Assessing Alterations in Vital Signs

Vital Sign	Normal Finding	Abnormal Finding
Temperature	Oral: 98.6°F (37°C) Axillary: 97.6°F (36.5–36.6°C) Rectal: 99.6°F (37.4–37.5°C)	Fever (temperature >101°F [38.3°C] in an adult)
Pulse	50 to 100 beats/minute in a regular and strong pattern	Tachycardia (>100 beats/minute)
		Bradycardia (<60 beats/minute)
Respiration	12 to 18 breaths/minute	Tachypnea (>24 breaths/minute)
		Bradypnea (<10 breaths/minute)
Blood pressure	120/80	Hypotension (<90 mm Hg systolic)
		Hypertension (>140 mm Hg systolic and/or 90 mm Hg diastolic)

Adapted from Ignativicius, D., Bayne, M. V. (1991). *Medical-surgical nursing: A nursing process approach* (p. 432). Philadelphia: W. B. Saunders.

puted tomography, magnetic resonance imaging [MRI], ultrasonography, biopsies and aspirations such as liver biopsy and bone marrow aspiration, endoscopic procedures such as colonoscopy, esophagoscopy, and duodenoscopy)

Assessing the Patient for Allergies and Hypersensitivity Reactions

- Ask the patient about allergies or hypersensitivity reactions to tape, iodine products, narcotics, antibiotics, local anesthetics, and other drugs.

Possible Indication	Possible Postoperative Complication
Infection	Systemic infection
Dehydration (when accompanied by decreased skin turgor)	Wound infection, dehiscence, or evisceration
	Fluid imbalance
Pain	Shock
Fever	Poor tissue perfusion
Dehydration	Vascular collapse
Anemia	Cardiac arrhythmias
Hypoxia	Renal failure
Shock	Anesthetic complications
Drug effects (e.g., of digitalis)	Spinal shock
Spinal injury	Increased intracranial pressure (see also complications for tachycardia)
Head injury	
Atelectasis	Tissue hypoxia
Pneumonia	Anesthetic complications
Pain or anxiety	Pneumonia
Pleurisy	Atelectasis
Infection	
Renal failure	
Brain lesion	See complications for tachypnea
Respiratory center depression	Poor tissue perfusion
Shock	Renal failure
Myocardial infarction	Vasodilation
Hemorrhage	Shock
Spinal injury	
Anxiety or pain	Stroke
Renal disease	Hemorrhage
Coronary artery disease	Myocardial infarction

- If the patient reports allergies or hypersensitivity reactions to food or chemical substances, determine the type of foods or substances and the type of reaction experienced.
- A history of anaphylaxis, asthma, or other respiratory difficulties related to the presence of allergens, toxins, or antigens should be noted and communicated to the anesthetist (Table 5).

Assessing the Patient's Nutritional Status (Table 6)

- Check for the presence of teeth.
- Look at the patient's fluid and electrolyte status.

Text continued on p. 14.

TABLE 2
Common Preoperative Blood Tests

Test	Normal Range
Potassium	3.5–5 mEq/L
Sodium	136–145 mEq/L
Chloride	96–106 mEq/L
Carbon dioxide	22–34 mEq/L
Glucose (fasting)	60–100 mg/dl
White blood cell count	4500–11,000 cells/mm³
Hemoglobin	12–15 g/dl (women)
	14–16.5 g/dl (men)
Hematocrit	37–45% (women)
	42–50% (men)
Creatinine	0.6–1 mg/dl (women)
	0.8–1.7 mg/dl (men)
Blood urea nitrogen	5–15 mg/dl
Prothrombin time	12–14 s (2–2.5 times normal is a therapeutic range)
Partial thromboplastin time	28–44 s (results are compared with aging laboratory control)

Adapted from Ignativicius, D., Bayne, M. V. (1991). *Medical-surgical nursing: A nursing process approach* (pp. 435–437). Philadelphia: W. B. Saunders.

Abnormal Findings	
Increase	**Decrease**
Dehydration	Excessive use of diuretics
Renal failure	Nausea, vomiting, hypotension, malnutrition, cardiac arrhythmias
Cardiac or renal failure	Nasogastric drainage
Hypertension	Vomiting, diarrhea
Excess amounts of intravenous fluids containing normal saline	Excessive use of laxatives and/or diuretics
Edema	
Alkalosis	Excessive nasogastric drainage
Dehydration	Vomiting
Renal failure	Excessive use of diuretics
Chronic obstructive pulmonary disease	Hyperventilation
Respiratory acidosis	Diabetic acidosis
Intestinal obstruction	Diarrhea
Vomiting or nasogastric suctioning	
Hyperglycemia	Hypoglycemia
Excess amounts of intravenous fluids containing glucose	
Pancreatic and/or hepatic disease	
Infection	Immune deficit
Fluid overload	Dehydration
	Excessive blood loss
	Anemia
Renal damage with destruction of large number of nephrons	Atrophy of muscle tissue
Dehydration	Overhydration
Renal failure	Liver failure
Excessive protein in diet	Malnutrition
Coagulation defect	Increased chance of embolus (thromboplebitis, pulmonary emboli)
Increased chance of hemorrhage	
Too high a dose of anticoagulant (aspirin, heparin, warfarin)	

TABLE 3

Normal Findings in Common Preoperative Blood Tests for Pediatric Patients

Test	Normal Range	
Potassium (mmol/L)	Newborn:	3.9–5.9
	Infant:	4.1–5.3
	Child:	3.4–4.7
	Thereafter:	3.5–5.1
Sodium (mmol/L)	Newborn:	134–146
	Infant:	139–146
	Child:	138–145
	Thereafter:	136–146
Chloride (mmol/L)	Cord:	96–104
	Newborn:	97–110
	Thereafter:	98–106
Carbon dioxide (mmol/L)	Cord:	14–22
	Premature:	14–27
	Newborn:	13–22
	Infant:	20–28
	Child:	20–28
	Thereafter:	23–30
Glucose (fasting) (mg/dl)	Cord:	45–96
	Premature:	20–60
	Neonate:	30–60
	Newborn,	
	1 d:	40–60
	>1 d:	50–90
	Child:	60–100
	Adult:	70–105
Creatinine (mg/dl)	Cord:	0.6–1.2
	Newborn:	0.3–1
	Infant:	0.2–0.4
	Child:	0.3–0.7
	Adolescent:	0.5–1.0
	Adult,	
	Male:	0.6–1.2
	Female:	0.5–1.1
Blood urea nitrogen (mg/dl)	Cord:	21–40
	Premature	
	(1 wk):	3–25
	Newborn:	3–12
	Infant or child:	5–18
	Thereafter:	7–18
Prothrombin time (s)	In general:	11–15
	(varies with type of thromboplastin)	
	Newborn:	prolonged by 2–3

Adapted from Behrman, R. E., Vaughan, V. C. (eds) (1987). *Nelson Textbook of Pediatrics* (13th ed). (pp. 1536–1538). Philadelphia: W. B. Saunders.

Test	Normal Range	
Partial thromboplastin time	Premature (48 h):	7.35–7.5
	Birth, full term:	7.11–7.36
	5–10 min:	7.09–7.3
	30 min:	7.21–7.38
	>1 h:	7.26–7.49
	1 d:	7.29–7.45
	Thereafter:	7.35–7.45
	Must be corrected for body temperature	
White blood cell count (1000 cells/mm³ [ul])	Birth:	9–30
	24 h:	9.4–34
	1 mo:	5–19.5
	1–3 y:	6–17.5
	4–7 y:	5.5–15.5
	8–13 y:	4.5–13.5
	Adult:	4.5–11
Hemoglobin (g/dl)	1–3 d (capillary):	14.5–22.5
	2 mo:	0.9–14.
	6–12 y:	11.5–15.5
	12–18 y,	
	Male:	13–16
	Female:	12–16
	18–49 y,	
	Male:	13.5–17.5
	Female:	12–16
Hematocrit (% of packed red blood cells)	1 d (capillary):	48–69
	2 d:	48–75
	3 d:	44–72
	2 mo:	28–42
	6–12 y:	35–45
	12–18 y,	
	Male:	37–49
	Female:	36–46
	18–49 y,	
	Male:	41–53
	Female:	36–46

TABLE 4
Common Preoperative Urine Chemistry Values

Characteristic/Component	Normal Finding
Color	Pale yellow
Odor	Specific aromatic odor, similar to that of ammonia
Turbidity	Clear
Specific gravity	Usually 1.015–1.025; possible range 1.01–1.03
pH	6; possible range 4.6–8
Glucose	None or <15 mg/dl
Ketones	None
Protein	2–8 mg/100 ml
Red blood cells	1 or 2 per high-power field
White blood cells	1 to 3 per high-power field
Bilirubin	None
Casts	A few or none, composed of red or white blood cells, protein, or tubular cell casts
Crystals	None
Bacteria	<1000 colonies/ml
Creatinine (clearance)	0.8–2 g/24 h Males: 1–2 g/24 h Females: 0.6–1.8 g/24 h
Urea nitrogen	6–17 g/24 h
Sodium	40–180 mEq/24 h
Chloride	110–254 mEq/24 h
Calcium	50–300 mg/24 h
Total catecholamines	110–254 mEq/24 h

From Ignativicius, D., Bayne, M. V. (1991). *Medical-surgical nursing: A nursing process approach* (pp. 1816, 1819). Philadelphia: W. B. Saunders.

Significance of Abnormal Finding

Dark amber indicates concentrated urine.

Pale yellow indicates dilute urine.

Dark red or brown indicates blood in the urine; brown also may indicate increased urinary bilirubin level.

Other color changes may result from diet or medications.

Foul smell indicates possible infection and/or dehydration.

Cloudy urine indicates infection or sediment.

Changes reflect a disturbance in the concentrating and diluting function of the tubules. Specific gravity may become fixed in renal insufficiency.

Changes are caused by diet, medications, infection, acid-base imbalance, and altered renal function.

Presence may indicate decreased tubular reabsorption capacity or hyperglycemia that exceeds this capacity.

Presence reflects incomplete metabolism of fatty acids, as in diabetes mellitus.

Increased levels may indicate stress, infection, strenuous exercise, or glomerular disorders.

Increased levels are normal with indwelling or intermittent catheterization or menses, but may reflect tumor, stones, or glomerular disorders.

Increased levels may indicate infectious or inflammatory processes.

Presence suggests hepatic or biliary disease or obstruction.

Increased levels indicate presence of bacteria or protein, which is seen in severe renal disease.

Presence or normal and/or abnormal crystals may indicate that the specimen has been allowed to stand.

Increased levels indicate need for urine culture to determine the presence of urinary tract infection.

Increased levels indicate glomerular dysfunction caused by renal disease, shock, or hypovolemia.

Increased levels commonly result from high-protein diet, dehydration, trauma, or sepsis.

Decreased levels are seen in hemorrhage, shock, and hyperaldosteronism.

Increased levels are common with diuretic therapy, excessive salt intake, and hypokalemia.

Decreased levels are seen in certain renal diseases.

Increased levels are commonly seen with calcium renal stones and hypercalcemia.

Decreased levels indicate hypocalcemia.

Increased levels occur with hypertension, pheochromocytoma, neuroblastomas, stress, or strenuous exercise.

TABLE 5

Most Common Agents That Cause Anaphylaxis

Drugs/Foreign Proteins
Antibiotics: penicillin, cephalosporins, tetracycline, sulfonamides,
    streptomycin, vancomycin, chloramphenicol, amphotericin B, and others
Adrenocorticotropic hormone, insulin, vasopressin, protamine
Allergen extracts, muscle relaxants, hydrocortisone, vaccines
Local anesthetics: lidocaine, procaine
Whole blood, cryoprecipitate, immune serum globulin
Radiocontrast media
Opiates

Foods
Shellfish
Eggs
Legumes, nuts
Grains
Berries
Preservatives

Insects/Animals
Hymenoptera: bees, wasps, hornets
Fire ants
Snake venom

Other Agents
Pollens
Exercise
Heat/cold
Other agents

From Ignativicius, D., Bayne, M. V. (1991). *Medical-surgical nursing: A nursing process
    approach* (p. 654). Philadelphia: W. B. Saunders.

- Determine the presence of acute gastrointestinal disorders, such
  as vomiting and diarrhea, which may result in a serious imbalance of fluids and electrolytes.
- Evaluate the patient's weight for signs of alteration in nutrition
  (more or less than body requirements).
- Review fluid intake and output.

Nutritional assessment data provide clues for identifying alterations
in the nutritional-metabolic pattern. Potential nursing diagnoses include the following:

- Alteration in nutrition: more than body requirements
- Alteration in nutrition: less than body requirements
- High risk for impaired wound healing

Assessing the Patient's Integumentary System

(Ignatavicius and Bayne, 1991, pp. 1140–1151)

- Determine whether the patient's family has a chronic tendency toward skin disorders.
- Ask if there have been recent complaints with skin problems. If the patient has existing skin problems, determine when the problems began.
- If a skin problem exists, determine whether it is associated with itching, burning, stinging, numbness, pain, fever, nausea and vomiting, diarrhea, sore throat, cold, stiff neck, exposure to new foods, new soaps or cosmetics, new clothing or bed linens, or stressful situations.
- Describe what makes the skin problem worse and what makes it better.
- When assessing the patient for allergies or reactions to toxic substances, determine whether there have been skin reactions.
- Ask the patient his or her occupation and whether he or she is exposed to irritants.
- Review nutritional assessment data.
- Observe the patient's skin color, temperature, and texture (Table 7).
- Check the patient's skin for lesions (Table 8).
- Check the patient's nails (Table 9).
- Look for signs of edema.
- Examine the patient's skin for moisture content.

Integumentary assessment data provide clues for identifying alterations in the nutritional-metabolic pattern. Potential nursing diagnoses include the following:

- High risk for impaired skin integrity
- Impaired skin integrity
- Impaired tissue integrity

Assessing the Patient's Cardiovascular System

(Melonakos, 1990, pp. 26–28)

- Ask the patient if she or he has experienced progressive weakness, shortness of breath, syncope, diaphoresis, nausea, or vomiting. If the patient has had these symptoms, ask under what circumstances they occurred.
- Determine whether the patient has a history of heart disease. If so, ask what type of heart disease.
- Ask the patient if family members have experienced heart disease, diabetes, stroke, and thromboembolism.
- Explore the type of medications the patient takes for existing cardiovascular disease, such as nitroglycerin, digitalis, diuretics, antihypertensives, and potassium supplements.

Text continued on p. 20.

TABLE **6**
Physical Signs of Malnutrition

Body Area	Normal Appearance
Hair	Shiny; firm; not easily plucked
Face	Skin color uniform; smooth, pink, healthy appearance; not swollen
Eyes	Bright, clear, shiny; no sores at corners of eyelids; membranes healthy pink and moist. No prominent blood vessels or mound of tissue on sclera
Lips	Smooth, not chapped or swollen
Tongue	Deep red in appearance; not swollen or smooth
Teeth	No cavities; no pain; bright
Gums	Healthy; red; do not bleed; not swollen
Glands	Face not swollen
Skin	No signs of rashes, swellings, dark or light spots
Nails	Firm, pink
Muscular and skeletal systems	Good muscle tone; some fat under skin; can walk or run without pain
Internal systems:	
Cardiovascular	Normal heart rate and rhythm; no murmurs or abnormal rhythms; normal blood pressure for age
Gastrointestinal	No palpable organs or masses (in children, however, liver edge may be palpable)
Nervous	Psychological stability; normal reflexes

From Nutrition assessment in health programs, part I—Methodology, clinical assessment of nutrition status. (1973). *American Journal of Public Health, 63* (Suppl.), 18.

Signs Associated With Malnutrition

Lack of natural shine; hair dull and dry; thin and sparse; hair fine, silky, and straight, color changes (flag sign); can be easily plucked

Skin color loss (depigmentation); skin dark over cheeks and under eyes (malar and supraorbital pigmentation); lumpiness or flakiness of skin of nose and mouth; swollen face; enlarged parotid glands; scaling of skin around nostrils (nasolabial seborrhea)

Eye membranes are pale (pale conjunctivae); redness of membranes (conjunctival injection); Bitot spots; redness and fissuring of eyelid corners (angular palpebritis); dryness of eye membranes (conjunctival xerosis); cornea has dull appearance (corneal xerosis); cornea is soft (keratomalacia); scar on cornea; ring of fine blood vessels around corner (circumcorneal injection)

Redness and swelling of mouth or lips (cheilosis), especially at corners of mouth (angular fissures and scars)

Swelling; scarlet and raw tongue; magenta (purplish) color of tongue; smooth tongue; swollen sores; hyperemic and hypertrophic papillae; and atrophic papillae

May be missing or erupting abnormally; gray or black spots (fluorosis); cavities (caries)

"Spongy" and bleed easily; recession of gums

Thyroid enlargement (front and neck); parotid enlargement (cheeks become swollen)

Dryness of skin (xerosis); sandpaper feel of skin (follicular hyperkeratosis); flakiness of skin; skin swollen and dark; red, swollen pigmentation of exposed areas (pellagrous dermatosis); excessive lightness or darkness of skin (dyspigmentation); black and blue maks due to skin bleeding (petechiae); lack of fat under skin

Nails are spoon shaped (koilonychia); brittle, ridged nails

Muscles have "wasted" appearance; baby's skull bones are thin and soft (craniotabes); round swelling of front and side of head (frontal and parietal bossing); swelling of ends of bones (epiphyseal enlargement); small bumps on both sides of chest wall (on ribs)—beading of ribs; baby's soft spot on head does not harden at proper time (persistently open anterior fontanelle); knock-knees or bowlegs; bleeding into muscle (musculoskeletal hemorrhages); person cannot get up or walk properly

Rapid heart rate (above 100 beats/minute tachycardia); enlarged heart; abnormal rhythm; elevated blood pressure

Liver enlargement; enlargement of spleen (usually indicates other associated diseases)

Mental irritability and confusion; burning and tingling of hands and feet (paresthesia); loss of position and vibratory sense; weakness and tenderness of muscles (may result in inability to walk); decrease and loss of ankle and knee reflexes

TABLE 7
Assessing the Integument

Alteration	Cause
White skin color (pallor)	Decreased hemoglobin level Decreased blood flow to the skin (vasoconstriction)
Yellow-orange skin color	Genetically determined defect of the melanocyte (decreased pigmentation) Acquired patchy loss of pigmentation Increased total serum bilirubin level (jaundice) Increased serum carotene level (carotenemia) Increased urochrome level
Red skin color (erythema)	Increased blood flow to the skin (vasodilation)
Blue skin color	Increase in deoxygenated blood (cyanosis)
Reddish blue skin color	Bleeding from vessels in tissue: Petechiae (1–3 mm) Ecchymosis (>3 mm) Increased overall amount of hemoglobin Decreased peripheral circulation
Brown skin color	Increased melanin production Café au lait spots (tan-brown patches) <6 spots >6 spots Melanin and hemosiderin deposits (bronze or grayish tan color)

From Ignatavicius, D., Bayne, M. V. (1991). *Medical-surgical nursing: A nursing process approach* (pp. 1142, 1147). Philadelphia: W. B. Saunders.

Location	Significance
Conjunctivae	Anemia
Mucous membranes	Shock or blood loss
Nail beds	Chronic vascular compromise
Palms and soles	Sudden emotional upset
Lips	Edema
Generalized	Albinism
Localized	Vitiligo; tinea versicolor
Generalized	Increased hemolysis of red blood cells
Mucous membranes	
Sclera	Liver disorders
Perioral	Increased ingestion of carotene-containing foods
Palms and soles	Pregnancy
Absent in sclera and mucous membranes	Thyroid deficiency
	Diabetes
Generalized	Chronic renal failure (uremia)
Absent in sclera and mucous membranes	
Generalized	Generalized inflammation
Localized	Localized inflammation (sunburn, cellulitis, trauma, and rashes)
Face, cheeks, nose, and upper chest	Fever; increased alcohol intake
Area of exposure	Exposure to cold
Nail beds	Cardiopulmonary disease
Mucous membranes	
Generalized	Methemoglobinemia
Localized	Thrombocytopenia
	Increased blood vessel fragility
Generalized	Polycythemia vera
Localized (to area of involvement)	Chronic inflammation
Pressure points, areolae, palmar creases, and genitalia	Exposure to sunlight
	Addison disease
Face, areolae, vulva, and linea nigra	Pregnancy; oral contraceptives (melasma)
Localized	Nonpathogenic
Generalized	Neurofibromatosis
Distal lower extremities	Chronic venous stasis
Exposed areas or generalized	Hemochromatosis

Continued.

Table 7
Assessing the Integument–Continued

Alteration	Cause
Localized edema Dependent or pitting edema	Inflammatory response Fluid and electrolyte imbalance Venous and cardiac insufficiency
Nonpitting edema	Endocrine imbalance
Increased moisture	Autonomic nervous system stimulation
Decreased moisture	Dehydration Endocrine imbalance
Increased temperature	Increased blood flow to skin
Decreased temperature	Decreased blood flow to skin
Decreased turgor	Decreased elasticity of dermis (tenting when pinched)
Rough or thick skin	Irritation, friction Sun damage Excessive collagen production
Soft or smooth skin	Endocrine disturbances

- Assess the patient's social history. Look for occupation-related stress, type A behavior patterns, stress related to marital or family status, and recent stressful life events.
- Determine the patient's smoking and alcohol habits and the amount of caffeine intake.
- Review nutritional assessment data, particularly typical eating patterns and salt intake.
- Assess the patient's activity level. Ask about exercise patterns and participation in cardiac rehabilitation activities.
- Assess the patient's pulse, including rate, amplitude, deficits, and peripheral pulses (Table 10).
- Assess the cardiac area for pulsations or other abnormalities (Table 11).
- Look for distended neck veins. The veins should distend only if

Location	Significance
Area of injury or involvement	Trauma
Ambulatory: dorsum of foot and medial ankle	Congestive heart failure
	Renal disease
Bedridden: buttocks, sacrum, and lower back	Hepatic cirrhosis
	Venous thrombosis or stasis
Generalized, but more easily seen over the tibia	Hypothyroidism (myxedema)
Face, axillae, skin folds, palms, and soles	Fever, anxiety, activity
	Hyperthyroidism
Buccal mucous membranes with progressive involvement of other skin surfaces	Postmenopause
	Hypothyroidism
	Normal aging
Generalized	Fever, hypermetabolic states
Localized	Inflammation
Generalized	Impending shock, sepsis, anxiety
	Hypothyroidism
Localized	Interference with vascular flow
Abdomen, forehead, or radial aspect of wrist	Sever dehydration
	Sudden severe weight loss
	Normal aging
Pressure points (soles, palms, and elbows)	Calluses
	Chronic eczema
	Atopic skin diseases
Areas of sun exposure	Normal aging
Localized or generalized	Scleroderma
	Keloids
Generalized	Hyperthyroidism

the patient lowers the head to assume the supine position. They should not distend if the patient remains in the sitting position.

- Check the patient for cardiomegaly. It is present if the apex of the heart is percussed past the midclavicular line.
- Palpate for thrills or murmurs over heart valve areas (aortic, pulmonic, tricuspid, and mitral).
- Check the patient for pitting edema. Use the 1+, 2+, 3+, or 4+ scale to describe the severity of edema.
- Assess the patient for cold or pale feet, absent or diminished peripheral pulses, cyanosis or flushing of the extremities, and leg cramps on walking. Pay particular attention to leg and foot care in the postoperative period in any patient who demonstrates one or more of these symptoms.
- Review laboratory values (Table 12).

Table **8**

Risk Factors For Altered Skin Integrity in the Elderly

Factor	Implications
Dermal Ulcers	
Increased likelihood of immobility	Increased potential for injury and trauma
	Increased likelihood of pressure sores
Increased incidence of peripheral vascular disease	Increased potential for ischemic ulcers (e.g., arterial ulcers)
	Increased potential for venous insufficiency
Increased prevalence of nutritional deficiency	Prolonged wound healing
	Reduced immunocompetence
Increased prevalence of peripheral neuropathy	Increased potential for injury or trauma
Increased prevalence of cerebellar dysfunction	Same
Rashes	
Increased drug use	Increased potential for allergic or toxic drug reactions
Increased incidence of herpes zoster	
Decreased immunocompetence	Increased potential for superinfection of rash
Increased prevalence of dry skin	Decreased protection against chemical irritants
Increased incidence of incontinence	Increased exposure to chemical irritants (e.g., urine)

From Matteson, M. A., McConnell, E. S. (1988). *Gerontological nursing: Concepts and practice.* Philadelphia: W. B. Saunders.

- Evaluate the outcomes of angiography, scans, stress testing, pulmonary function tests, x-ray studies, fluoroscopy, and other diagnostic tests (Table 13).

Cardiovascular assessment data provide clues for identifying alterations in the activity-exercise pattern. Potential nursing diagnoses include the following:

- High risk for activity intolerance
- Activity intolerance
- Decreased cardiac output
- Altered tissue perfusion

Assessing the Patient's Respiratory System (Melonakos, 1990, pp. 20–23)

- If the patient reports episodes of shortness of breath, ask when they occur.
- Evaluate the patient for the presence of a cough. If a cough is

TABLE **9**
Assessing Nail Color

Alteration	Clinical Findings	Significance
White	Horizontal white banding or areas of opacity	Chronic hepatic or renal disease (hypoalbuminemia)
	Generalized pallor of nail bed	Shock
		Anemia
		Early arteriosclerotic changes (toenails)
		Myocardial infarction
Yellow-brown	Diffuse yellow to brown discoloration	Jaundice
		Peripheral lymphedema
		Bacterial or fungal infection of the nail
		Psoriasis
		Diabetes
		Cardiac failure
		Staining from tobacco, nail polish, or dyes
		Chronic tetracycline therapy
		Normal aging (yellow-gray color)
	Vertical brown banding extending from the proximal nail fold distally	Normal finding in black patients
		Nevus or melanoma of nail matrix in Caucasian patients
Red	Thin, dark red vertical lines 1–3 mm in length (splinter hemorrhages)	Bacterial endocarditis
		Trichinosis
		Trauma to nail bed
		Normal finding in some patients
	Red discoloration of lunula	
	Dark red nail beds	Cardiac insufficiency
		Polycythemia vera
Blue	Diffuse blue discoloration that blanches with pressure	Respiratory failure
		Methemoglobinuria
		Venous stasis disease (toenails)

From Ignatavicius, D., Bayne, M. V. (1991). *Medical-surgical nursing: A nursing process approach* (p. 1149). Philadelphia: W. B. Saunders.

present, determine whether it is productive, hacking, paroxysmal, brassy, habitual, or nervous.

- Explore the patient's medical history for episodes of respiratory disease. If present, determine the type of therapy prescribed and the effectiveness of treatment.

TABLE **10**

Assessing Pulse

Measurement

Place first, second, and third fingers on the patient's radial artery to determine the radial pulse.

Evaluate rate, rhythm, and amplitude.

Count the radial pulse for 30 s and multiply by 2.

If irregularities are noted, take an apical pulse for 1 min.

Normal pulse rate is 60–80 beats/min for an average adult.

Pulse Rhythm

Normal dysrhythmias

  The pulse rate speeds up at the end of inspiration and slows down with expiration in young adults and children.

  Occasional premature beats are normal.

Abnormal dysrhythmias

  Pulse deficit exists if the apical rate differs from the radial rate.

Pulse Amplitude

Pulse amplitude refers to the measurement of pulse force or strength.

Amplitude

  3+ = bounding pulse

  2+ = normal pulse

  1+ = weak, thready pulse

  0 = absent pulse

Bounding pulse implies a widened pulse pressure, which is the difference between the systolic and diastolic pressures.

Weak, thready pulse implies a narrowed pulse pressure.

Pulse Points

Obtain peripheral pulses for patients undergoing angiography or cardiac or vascular surgery.

Peripheral pulses include radial, ulnar, brachial, femoral, popliteal, dorsalis pedis, and posterior tibilalis.

Data from Melonakos, K. (1990). *Saunders pocket reference for nurses* (pp. 10–12). Philadelphia: W. B. Saunders.

- If the patient engages in an exercise program, determine whether breathing exercises are part of the program.
- Check the patient's chest symmetry on inspiration.
- Look for abnormalities such as barrel-, funnel-, or pigeon-shaped chest and spinal deformities.
- Evaluate the patient's skin for mottling, scars, irregularities, and odor.
- Assess the patient's respiratory pattern, including rate and rhythm. Watch the patient breathe to determine the presence of

TABLE 11
Abnormal Heart Sounds

Sound	Description	Cause
Quiet or muffled heart sounds		Thick chest wall, severe overload, cardiac tamponade
Gallops	Extra heart sounds best heard over apex	Cardinal sign of congestive heart failure
Snaps and clicks	High-pitched sounds usually associated with murmurs	Rapid displacement of a valve from high pressure due to stenosis
Murmurs	High- or low-pitched sounds	Turbulent blood flow through a valve due to congenital or acquired defects
Friction rub	A sound like two pieces of leather rubbing together	Associated with pericarditis

Adapted from Melonakos, K. (1990). *Saunders pocket reference for nurses* (p. 11). Philadelphia: W. B. Saunders.

TABLE 12
Using Laboratory Values to Assess Cardiovascular Status

Parameter	Assessment
Complete blood count	Check WBC, hemoglobin level, and hematocrit to identify infectious or anemic trends.
Electrolytes	Check potassium to determine if the patient is receiving diuretics or potassium supplements.
Blood gases	Check pH, oxygen pressure, and bicarbonate level for normal limits.
Cardiac enzymes	Check for trends in elevation of creatine kinase, lactate dehydrogenase, aspartate aminotransferase (formerly known as serum glutamic-oxaloacetic transaminase), and isoenzyme studies.
Coagulation studies	Check prothrombin time for oral coagulants, partial thromboplastin time for heparin therapy.
Urinalysis	Check specific gravity and look for presence of protein.
Blood urea nitrogen	Check kidney function.
Serum drug levels	Check for presence of digitalis, lidocaine, procainamide, and quinidine.

Data from Melonakos, K. (1990). *Saunders pocket reference for nurses* (pp. 28–29, 726). Philadelphia: W. B. Saunders.

TABLE **13**

Physiologic Cardiovascular Changes With Aging

Resting
Heart rate–unchanged
Left ventricular stroke volume– ↑
Cardiac output– ↓
Left ventricular end-diastolic pressure–unchanged
Ejection time– ↑
Systolic blood pressure– ↑
Systemic vascular resistance– ↑

Exercise
Maximal heart rate– ↓
Maximal oxygen consumption– ↓
Arteriovenous oxygen difference– ↓
Maximal cardiac output– ↓
Left ventricular end-diastolic pressure– ↑
Systolic blood pressure– ↑
Systemic vascular resistance– ↑

Adapted from Schrier, R. (1982). *Clinical internal medicine in the aged.* Philadelphia: W. B. Saunders.

    pursed-lip breathing, nasal flaring, chest breathing versus abdominal breathing, retractions, or splinting because of pain.
- Review laboratory results, especially complete blood count, electrolyte values, hematocrit, and hemoglobin concentration.
- If indicated, carefully evaluate blood gas results for abnormalities.
- Review diagnostic studies and note and communicate to the physician abnormal results, especially abnormal findings of radiography, electrocardiography, biopsies, fluid aspirations, lung scans, pulmonary function studies, and bronchoscopy (Tables 14 to 20).

TABLE **14**

Assessing Respirations

Assess the patient's respirations for rate and quality.
Count the rate for 30 s and multiply by 2. If respiratory or cardiac problems are identified, evaluate the respiratory rate for 60 s.
For the average adult, the normal respiratory rate is 16–20 breaths/min. A patient's rate varies depending on age, exercise, and environmental conditions. Normally, a patient takes 3 deep breaths/min.

Data from Melonakos, K. (1990). *Saunders pocket reference for nurses* (p. 12). Philadelphia: W. B. Saunders.

TABLE 15
Examining the Lungs

Palpation

Gently palpate the patient all over the thorax for any tender areas.

Check the patient's chest expansion by placing the hands on either side of the chest at the lung bases and ask the patient to inhale deeply. Look for equal expansion. The hands should move equally upward and slightly outward.

Assess the patient for tactile fremitus by palpating for vibrations on the chest wall when the patient says "ninety-nine." A decreased fremitus may indicate pneumothorax or pleural effusion. Increased fremitus may indicate consolidation secondary to atelectasis or pneumonia.

Percussion

Dullness on percussion may indicate consolidation, atelectasis, or effusion.

Hyperresonance on percussion may indicate pneumothorax or chronic obstructive pulmonary disease.

Auscultation

Instruct the patient to cough and clear the upper airway. Next, have the patient breathe deeply through the mouth.

Start at the trachea and move in a zigzag pattern, auscultating the anterior, posterior, and lateral parts of the patient's thorax.

Listen for resonance, breath and voice sounds, rales and rhonchi, and friction rub.

Data from Melonakos, K. (1990). *Saunders pocket reference for nurses* (pp. 7, 22–23). Philadelphia: W. B. Saunders.

TABLE 16
Abnormal Breath Sounds

Breath Sounds	Characteristics	Indications
Rales	Sounds like fizzing seltzer; may be fine, medium, or coarse; wet or crackling	"Wet," pulmonary edema; "dry," pulmonary fibrosis
Rhonchi	Bubbling or rumbling sounds	Chronic bronchitis or any disorder with retained pulmonary secretions
Wheezing	Musical sounds, varied pitch	Asthma, chronic bronchitis, or any disorder reducing the caliber of airways
Pleural friction rub	Like a squeaky, groaning leather shoe	Pleurisy, pulmonary embolus

Data from Melonakos, K. (1990). *Saunders pocket reference for nurses* (p. 23). Philadelphia: W. B. Saunders.

TABLE 17

Effects of Aging on the Respiratory System

Respiratory Abnormality	Physiological Basis	Clinical Disorders
Decline in bellows function	Increased chest wall stiffness Loss of elastic recoil Decreased respiratory muscle strength Increased airway collapsibility	"Senile" emphysema
Abnormal gas exchange	Ventilation-perfusion mismatch Reduced diffusing for carbon monoxide	Arterial hypoxemia
	Increased alveolar-arterial oxygen gradient	Decreased exercise tolerance
Abnormal breathing pattern	Diminished responsiveness to hypoxemia and hypercarbia	Cheyne-Stokes breathing
	Changing set point for ventilation due to fluctuating level of wakefulness	Periodic breathing
Upper airway obstruction	Decreased airway muscle tone due to loss of wakefulness stimulus, decreased metabolic respiratory drive	Snoring, sleep apnea, hypopnea, oxygen desaturation
Altered lung host-defense	Decreased ciliary action Impaired cough mechanism Decreased IgA production ?Decreased phagocytic function of alveolar macrophages	Increased susceptibility to infection (pneumonia and chronic bronchitis)

From Schrier, R. W. (1982). *Clinical internal medicine in the aged.* Philadelphia: W. B. Saunders.

Respiratory assessment data provide clues for identifying alterations in the activity-exercise pattern. Potential nursing diagnoses include the following:

- Ineffective airway clearance
- Ineffective breathing pattern
- Impaired gas exchange

Assessing the Patient's Gastrointestinal System
(Melonakos, 1990, pp. 29–33)

- Assess the patient for gastrointestinal pain.
- Assess for the presence of nausea, vomiting, and diarrhea.

- Determine when episodes of gastrointestinal distress occur, such as before or after meals. Search for precipitating factors, such as emotional stress, medications, specific foods, treatments, and exercise.
- If the patient reports vomiting or diarrhea, describe the frequency, amount, color, odor, and consistency.
- Assess the patient for constipation. Determine the time of the last bowel movement. Ask if laxatives or enemas were used.
- Assess the patient for episodes of belching, gas, and flatulence. Determine their frequency.
- Determine whether the patient has episodes of gastrointestinal bleeding. If so, describe the type of bleeding.
- Ask the patient about recent weight gain or loss.
- Determine whether the patient has a history of gastrointestinal problems. If so, inquire about the type of therapy used and whether it was effective.
- Ask whether the patient has experienced gastrointestinal problems related to allergies.
- Determine and list all medications the patient uses for gastrointestinal problems, such as over-the-counter antacids, laxatives, and sodium bicarbonate.
- Determine bowel and bladder habits and whether there has been a recent change in habits.
- Observe the patient's skin color and hair distribution.
- Look for jaundice.
- Inspect the skin for rashes, striae, pigmentations, or surgical wounds.
- Assess the patient for asymmetry, masses, herniations, visible peristalsis, or pulsations.
- Look at the contour of the patient's abdomen and describe it in terms of obesity, flatness, distention, hollowness, and cachexia.
- Auscultate, percuss, and palpate the abdomen.
- Review laboratory results, especially complete blood count, electrolyte values, and blood urea nitrogen level.
- Review diagnostic studies and note and communicate to the physician abnormal reports, especially reports of common gastrointestinal studies such as barium enema and barium swallow examinations, endoscopy, nuclear scans, sigmoidoscopy, ultrasonography, and radiography (Tables 21 to 24).

Gastrointestinal assessment data provide clues for identifying alterations in the elimination pattern. Potential nursing diagnoses include the following:

- Constipation
- Diarrhea
- Bowel incontinence

TABLE **18**
Evaluating Blood Gases

Test	Value
pH	7.35–7.45
Arterial carbon dioxide pressure (pCO$_2$)	35–45 mm Hg
Oxygen pressure (pO$_2$)	75–100 mm Hg (dependent on age and altitude); above 500 mg while receiving 100% oxygen
Oxygen (O$_2$) saturation	95% or greater
Bicarbonate (HCO$_3$)	24–28 mEq/L

Adapted from Melonakos, K. (1990). *Saunders pocket reference for nurses* (p. 106). Philadelphia: W. B. Saunders.

TABLE **19**
Types of Sputum

Type of Sputum	Characteristics	Indications
Mucoid	Thin, clear	Early bronchitis
Mucopurulent	Thick, viscous, greenish color, frothy	Pneumonia, late bronchitis, tuberculosis
Purulent	Thick, viscous, yellowish, offensive smell	Lung abscess, advanced tuberculosis, bronchiectasis, pneumonia
Nummular	Mucopurulent with small semisolid masses that sink in water	Advanced tuberculosis
Rusty	Mucopurulent, rust tinged, viscous	Pneumonia
Prune juice	Dark brown, offensive smelling	Late pneumonia or gangrene of lung
Hemoptysis	Bright red and frothy	Cancer, tuberculosis, pneumonia, pulmonary embolism, mitral stenosis, or aneurysm rupturing into bronchial tubes

Adapted from Melonakos, K. (1990). *Saunders pocket reference for nurses* (p. 22). Philadelphia: W. B. Saunders.

Abnormal Findings	
Increased	Decreased
Alkalosis	Acidosis
Compensated metabolic alkalosis	Compensated metabolic acidosis
Respiratory acidosis	Respiratory alkalosis
Administration of high concentration of oxygen	Decreased cardiac output
	Chronic lung disease
Polycythemia	Decreased efficiency of the lungs
Oxygen administration	High altitude
	Lung diseases
Compensated respiratory acidosis	Compensated respiratory alkalosis
Metabolic alkalosis	Metabolic acidosis

Assessing the Musculoskeletal System (Ignatavicius and Bayne, 1991, pp. 721–724)

- Obtain information about the patient's previous illnesses and accidents related to the musculoskeletal system.
- Ask about traumatic incidents such as sprains and fractures. Note the date of traumatic incidents, even if they occurred years in the past.
- Explore the patient's family history. Osteoporosis is often seen in several family generations, and bone cancer tends to be genetically linked.
- Determine whether the patient has regular exposure to sunlight. Inadequate exposure predisposes the patient to bone and muscle tone loss.
- Ask the patient or a significant other to describe the patient's eating patterns. Calcium or protein deficiency predisposes the patient to bone and muscle tone loss.
- Determine whether the patient has adequate vitamin C intake. Inadequate intake inhibits bone and tissue healing.
- Note the patient's weight. Obese patients with musculoskeletal problems are at risk for respiratory and circulatory complications. Obesity also places excessive strain and stress on joints and bones, which may lead to fractures and cartilage degeneration.
- Determine the patient's occupation, which may place the patient at risk for musculoskeletal injury or health problems.
- Look for gross deformities or impairment by observing the patient's posture, gait, and mobility (Table 25).

TABLE 20
Abnormal Respiratory Patterns

Pattern	Characteristics	Indications
Tachypnea	Rapid and shallow breathing	Associated with fever, pneumonia, respiratory alkalosis, and salicylate poisoning
Bradypnea	Slowed but regular breathing	Associated with the use of opiates and alcohol, tumors, metabolic disorders, and conditions affecting the medulla oblongata
Hyperventilation or Kussmaul breathing	Increased rate and depth of breathing	Associated with renal failure and diabetic ketoacidosis
Apnea	Periodic absence of breathing	Caused by mechanical obstruction or conditions affecting the respiratory center
Cheyne-Stokes	Periods of apnea followed by breath of increasing depth	Caused by increased intracranial pressure, severe congestive heart failure, renal failure, meningitis, drug overdose, and cerebral anoxia
Biot fast	Uniformly deep respirations marked by abrupt pauses	Associated with head injury
Ataxic breathing	Completely chaotic and irregular breathing	Associated with severe brain stem damage

Adapted from Melonakos, K. (1990). *Saunders pocket reference for nurses* (pp. 12–13). Philadelphia: W. B. Saunders.

- Inspect the patient's muscle mass for size and symmetry. Look at tone, shape, and strength. Determine the grip strength by having the patient squeeze a sphygmomanometer bulb and record the level of pressure achieved.
- Assess the head and neck, the vertebral spine, and the upper and lower extremities (Table 26).
- Review laboratory studies, especially serum calcium, phosphorus, and phosphate levels, erythrocyte sedimentation rate, and serum muscle enzyme levels (Table 27).

TABLE **21**
Examining the Abdomen

Auscultation
Perform auscultation before percussion or palpation to avoid stimulating peristalsis.
Because bowel sounds are high pitched, use the diaphragm of the stethoscope.
Normal bowel sounds should be heard in all four quadrants every 5–20 s.
Evaluate abnormal findings.
   Hypoactive bowel sounds (less than one per minute) indicate paralytic ileus, peritonitis, obstruction, hemorrhage, post abdominal surgery, mesenteric infarct, or no food in the bowel.
   Hyperactive bowel sounds (continuous sounds) may occur with vomiting or diarrhea, above bowel obstruction, or after eating.
   Vascular sounds may indicate aneurysm, vascular disease, heart murmur, or liver disease.

Percussion
Percuss all four quadrants.
Listen for areas of dullness and tympany.
   Tympanic areas: large and small intestines
   Dull areas: liver, spleen, bladder, and gravid uterus

Palpation
Palpate lightly for areas of tenderness, masses, and involuntary guarding.
Palpate deeply for normal anatomy, enlarged structures, masses, and pain.
   Liver, spleen, pancreas, and urinary bladder are not normally palpable.
   The lower pole of the right kidney may be palpated. The left kidney, however, is not normally palpable, except occasionally in thin individuals.
   Aorta is often palpable at the epigastrium slightly left of the midline. Aorta feels like a long, thin, consistent, pulsatile mass. An enlarged area may indicate aneurysm.
Do not mistake normal structures (such as feces-filled colon, distended bladder, gravid uterus, aorta, and sacral promontory) for masses.
Techniques for assessment of abdominal fluid include flank bulging and fluid shift.

Data from Melonakos, K. (1990). *Saunders pocket reference for nurses* (pp. 32–33). Philadelphia: W. B. Saunders.

   • Review diagnostic studies such as radiography, tomography and xeroradiography, myelography, diskography, arthrography, computed tomography, and bone or muscle biopsies (Table 28).
   Musculoskeletal assessment data provide clues for identifying alterations in the activity-exercise pattern. Potential nursing diagnoses include the following:
   • High risk for injury related to musculoskeletal impairment

TABLE 22
Primary Causes of Abdominal Pain

Obstruction
Peritoneal irritation
Vascular insufficiency
Ulceration
Altered bowel motility
Nerve injury
Referred pain from an extraabdominal site
Emotional stress

Adapted from Melonakos, K. (1990). *Saunders pocket reference for nurses* (p. 29). Philadelphia: W. B. Saunders.

TABLE 23
Characteristics of Gastrointestinal Bleeding

Vomitus	Stool
Bright red	Bright red
Brown	Blood tinged
Coffee grounds	Dark and tarry
Blood tinged	Positive for occult blood
Positive for occult blood	

Data from Melonakos, K. (1990). *Saunders pocket reference for nurses* (p. 31). Philadelphia: W. B. Saunders.

- Impaired physical mobility
- Self-care deficit

Assessing the Patient's Urinary System (Ignatavicius and Bayne, 1991, pp. 1808–1811)

- Note the patient's age and sex. Some urinary tract disorders are related to the age or sex of the patient.
- Assess the patient's personal and family history. Ask the patient about a history of urinary tract infections or urologic surgery. Note any history of arthritis, hypertension, and diabetes mellitus.
- Review nutritional assessment data.
- Review the patient's medication history. Determine whether the patient has taken medications for chronic health problems such as diabetes mellitus, hypertension, cardiac disorders, hormone deficiencies, and arthritis.

TABLE 24
Examining the Rectum and Anus

Don protective gloves.
Place the patient in the lateral Sims' position.
Observe the skin and surface characteristics of the perianal area.
The perianal area should be smooth and clear with no tenderness, fissures, hemorrhoids, scars, ulcers, skin irritation, or rectal prolapse.
Palpate the perianal area for tenderness and masses.
With gloved, lubricated index finger, perform digital examination.
   Sphincter muscle should tighten evenly around the finger with minimal discomfort for the patient.
   The rectal wall should be a continuous, smooth surface with no areas of tenderness, tumors, lumps, or masses.

Data from Melonakos, K. (1990). *Saunders pocket reference for nurses* (p. 33). Philadelphia: W. B. Saunders.

TABLE 25
Assessing Posture, Gait, and Mobility

Posture
Evaluate the patient's body build and alignment when standing and walking.
Look for curvature of the spine.
   Lordosis
   Scoliosis
   Kyphosis
Inspect the extremities for length, shape, and symmetry.

Gait
Evaluate the patient's balance and steadiness.
Determine the patient's ease and length of stride.
Look for limp or other asymmetrical leg movements or deformities.
Determine the patient's need for ambulatory assistive devices.

Mobility
Assess the patient's ability to perform activities of daily living.
Determine the extent of range of motion by having the patient demonstrate active movement of major joints.

From Ignatavicius, D., Bayne, M. V. (1991). *Medical-surgical nursing: A nursing process approach* (p. 723). Philadelphia: W. B. Saunders.

TABLE **26**

Assessing the Skeletal System

Head and Neck

Inspect and palpate the skull for shape, symmetry, tenderness, and masses.

Evaluate the temporomandibular joints by palpating while the patient opens his or her mouth. Common abnormal findings are tenderness or pain, crepitus, and a spongy swelling caused by excessive synovium and fluid, which can be palpated.

Observe and palpate each vertebra in the neck.

Vertebral Spine

Observe and palpate the thoracic, lumbar, and sacral spine. Look for malalignment, tenderness, and inability to flex, extend, and rotate.

Check for discomfort in the lower back by placing both hands over the lumbosacral area and applying pressure with the thumbs to elicit tenderness.

Upper Extremities

Assess both extremities concurrently.

Starting with the shoulders and moving to the elbows and then the wrists, check for size, swelling, deformity, malalignment, tenderness or pain, and mobility.

Assess hand function by palpating the metacarpophalangeal, proximal interphalangeal, and distal interphalangeal joints. Compare the same digits on the right and left hands.

Determine range of motion for each joint.

Lower Extremities

Evaluate the hip joints by determining the degree of mobility.

Assess the knee joints with the patient in a sitting position with the knees flexed. Look for fluid accumulation, or effusion, and limitations in movement with accompanying pain.

Inspect the ankles and feet. Observe, palpate, and test each joint for range of motion.

Data from Ignatavicius, D., Bayne, M. V. (1991). *Medical-surgical nursing: A nursing process approach* (p. 723). Philadelphia: W. B. Saunders.

- Assess the patient's urinary patterns. Ask whether the patient has experienced changes in the color of the urine, the pattern of urination, and the ability to start or control urination.
- Determine whether the patient has had alterations in the appearance of the urine.
- Ask whether the patient has experienced oliguria, anuria, polyuria, hesitancy, dysuria, or urgency (Table 29).

- Determine whether the patient has episodes of urinary incontinence. If so, describe the situations that result in incontinence.
- Assess the general condition of the patient. Look at the skin. Determine whether there is a yellow tinge, rashes, ecchymoses, and other discoloration. Check the pedal, pretibial, presacral, and periorbital tissues, which are common sites of edema in renal disorders.
- Assess the patient's level of consciousness.
- Check the patient's gait and hand coordination, which may also be affected by the presence of renal disease.

Urinary system assessment data provide clues for identifying alterations in the nutritional-metabolic and elimination patterns. Potential nursing diagnoses include the following:

- High risk for fluid volume deficit
- Fluid volume deficit
- Fluid volume excess
- Altered patterns of urinary elimination
- Functional incontinence
- Stress incontinence
- Total incontinence

PSYCHOSOCIAL ASSESSMENT

The perioperative nurse/RNFA assesses the patient's and the family's psychosocial health status by determining the patient's and/or the family's knowledge level concerning the perioperative experience and ability to

- Adhere to prescribed therapeutic regimens
- Implement self-care activities
- Handle fear
- Deal with anticipatory anxiety
- Recognize and resolve a body image disturbance
- Grieve successfully
- Effectively cope with the stress associated with surgery.

Assessing the Patient's Knowledge Level Concerning the Perioperative Experience (Gordon, 1987a, p. 186)

- Determine whether the patient and the family can adequately recall information about past surgical or invasive procedure experiences or demonstrate misunderstanding, misinterpretation, or misconceptions.
- Assess whether the patient or the family has had difficulty with accurately following through with previous instructions.

Text continued on p. 42.

TABLE 27

Using Laboratory Studies for Musculoskeletal Assessment

Test	Normal Range (Adults)
Serum calcium level	8–10.5 mg/dl or 4.5–5.5 mEq/L
Serum phosphorus level	2.5–4 mg/dl
Alkaline phosphatase level	30–90 IU/L (slightly higher in elderly)
Erythrocyte sedimentation rate	Westergren method Males: 0–15 mm/h Females: 0–20 mm/h Wintrobe method Males: 0–9 mm/h Females: 0–25 mm/h
Serum muscle enzyme level creatine kinase (CK_3)	15–150 IU/L
Lactate dehydrogenase (LDH_4 and LDH_5)	60–150 IU/L
Aspartate aminotransferase (serum glutamic-oxaloacetic transaminase)	10–50 mU/ml (slightly lower in women)
Aldolase A	1.3–8.2 U/dl

From Ignatavicius, D., Bayne, M. V. (1991). *Medical-surgical nursing: A nursing process approach* (p. 725). Philadelphia: W. B. Saunders.

Interpreting Abnormal Ranges

Hypercalcemia
    Metastatic cancers of the bone
    Paget disease
    Bone fractures in healing stage
Hypocalcemia
    Osteoporosis
    Osteomalacia
Hyperphosphatemia
    Bone fractures in healing stage
    Bone tumors
    Acromegaly
Hypophosphatemia
    Osteomalacia
Elevations
    Metastatic cancers of the bone
    Paget disease
    Osteomalacia
Elevations
    Infection
    Inflammation
    Carcinoma
    Cell or tissue destruction

Elevations
    Muscle trauma
    Progressive muscular dystrophy
    Effects of electromyography
Elevations
    Skeletal muscle necrosis
    Extensive cancer
    Progressive muscular dystrophy
Elevations
    Skeletal muscle trauma
    Progressive muscular dystrophy
Elevations
    Polymyositis and dermatomyositis
    Muscular dystrophy

TABLE **28**
Diagnostic Studies of the Musculoskeletal System

Examination or Test	Purpose
Standard radiography	Visualize the skeleton and supporting structures
	Observe bone density, alignment, swelling, and intactness
	Determine condition of joints, including the size of the joint space, the smoothness of articular cartilage, and synovial swelling
	Determine soft tissue involvement
Tomography and xeroradiography	Tomography is helpful in musculoskeletal assessment because it produces planes, or slices, for focus and blurs the images of other structures
	Xeroradiography highlights the contrast between structures, allowing margins and edges to be clearly seen
Myelography	Visualize the vertebral column, intervertebral disks, spinal nerve roots, and blood vessels
Diskography	Visualize an intervertebral disk
Arthrography	Visualize a joint
Computed tomography	Detect musculoskeletal problems (used with or without contrast medium)
Bone biopsy	Confirm the presence of infection or neoplasm
Muscle biopsy	Diagnose muscle atrophy (as in muscular dystrophy) and inflammation (as in polymyositis)
Electromyography	Determine the electrical potential generated in an individual muscle
	Usually accompanied by nerve conduction studies
	Helpful in the diagnosis of neuromuscular, lower motor neuron, and peripheral nerve disorders
Bone scan	Radionuclide test used to detect tumors, arthritis, osteomyelitis, osteoporosis, vertebral compression fractures, and unexplained bone pain

Data from Ignatavicius, D., Bayne, M. V. (1991). *Medical-surgical nursing: A nursing process approach* (p. 726–731). Philadelphia: W. B. Saunders; and Melonakos, K. (1990). *Saunders pocket reference for nurses* (p. 154). Philadelphia: W. B. Saunders.

Method

Standard x-ray imaging

X-ray imaging with higher doses of radiation

Injection of a contrast medium into the subarachnoid space of the spine

Injection of a contrast medium directly into the target disk

X-ray imaging of a joint after injection of a contrast medium (air or solution) to enhance visualization

Scanner produces a narrow x-ray beam that examines body section from many different angles

A computer produces a three-dimensional picture of the structure being studied

Small tumors may not be detected without the use of oral or intravenous contrast medium

Collection of a bone specimen for microscopic examination via needle or open extraction

Collection of a muscle specimen for microscopic examination via needle or open extraction

Multiple needle electrodes, varying from 1.3 to 7.5 cm ($\frac{1}{2}$ to 3 inches), are inserted

The patient performs activities to measure muscle potential during minimal and maximal contractions

Nerve and muscle activity is recorded on an oscilloscope

When done in conjuction with nerve conduction studies, flat electrodes are placed along the nerve to be evaluated, and small doses of electrical current are passed via the electrodes to the nerve and muscle innervated. If the muscle contracts, nerve conduction is confirmed

The radioactive isotope technetium (^{99m}Tc) is injected intravenously for visualization of the entire skeleton

Continued.

TABLE 28
Diagnostic Studies of the Musculoskeletal System–Continued

Examination or Test	Purpose
Gallium scan	This test is similar to the bone scan but is more specific and sensitive in detecting bone problems
Indium imaging	Used primarily to detect bone infection
Magnetic resonance imaging	Identify problems with muscle, tendons, and ligaments
Ultrasonography	Detect soft tissue disorders such as masses and fluid accumulation

TABLE 29
Terms for Urinary Dysfunction

Oliguria	Decrease in urine output, specifically an output of 100–400 ml/24 h
Anuria	Absence of urine output, specifically less than 100 ml/24 h
Polyuria	Increase in urine output, usually greater than 1500 ml/24 h
Dysuria	Any discomfort associated with urination
Hesitancy	Difficulties in initiating the flow of urine
Urgency	Sensations experienced when there is a sudden need to urinate; may be associated with urinary incontinence
Renal colic	Severe or spasmodic pain associated with renal or ureteral irritation that radiates into the perineal area, groin, scrotum, or labia

From Ignatavicius, D., Bayne, M. V. (1991). *Medical-surgical nursing: A nursing process approach* (p. 1810). Philadelphia: W. B. Saunders.

- Determine whether the patient can adequately perform self-care skills.
- Look for signs that demonstrate inappropriate or exaggerated behaviors such as hysteria, hostility, or apathy.

Assessing the Patient's and Family's Ability to Adhere to Prescribed Therapeutic Regimen (Gordon, 1987a, p. 48)

- Assess the patient for a history of noncompliance with prescribed therapeutic regimens.

Method
Radioactive medium used is gallium citrate (^{67}Ga), which is administered 3 d before the test because of the slow absorption rate of the material
The patient's leukocytes are separated from a blood sample, tagged with indium (^{111}In), and injected intravenously. In acute bone infections (osteomyelitis), the tagged leukocytes accumulate and can be seen on scanning
The image is produced through the interaction of magnetic fields, radiowaves, and atomic nuclei showing hydrogen density. The lack of hydrogen ions in cortical bone makes it easily distinguishable from soft tissues
Use of sound waves to produce an image of the tissue being studied

- If the patient is unable to provide self-care, determine whether there is a family history of noncompliance with prescribed therapeutic regimens.
- Ask whether the patient has support systems in place (family, friends).
- If the patient is unable to provide self-care, determine whether the patient or the family denies the presence of illness.
- Determine whether the patient or the family perceives that recommended therapeutic regimens are ineffective.
- Assess whether the patient or the family understands the seriousness of the health problem or the risk factors associated with potential health problems.
- Determine whether the patient or the family perceives a lack of susceptibility to the complications associated with the health problem.
- Determine whether the patient or the family has sufficient knowledge or skills to implement the recommended therapeutic regimens.
- Ask whether the patient or the family has a plan for integrating therapeutic recommendations into daily routines.

Assessing the Patient's Ability to Implement Self-Care Activities (Gordon, 1987a, p. 132)

- Assess for the presence of chronic pain or discomfort.
- Assess for the presence of acute pain or discomfort after surgery.
- Determine whether the patient has uncompensated perceptual-cognitive impairment.

- Determine whether the patient is experiencing severe anxiety.
- Look for signs of depression.

Assessing the Presence of Fear in the Patient (Gordon, 1987a, p. 198)

- Determine whether the patient views surgery as the focus of threat or danger.
- Assess whether the patient has feelings of dread, nervousness, or concern about the surgical event.
- Listen for verbal clues that the patient expects danger to self during the perioperative period.
- Determine whether the patient has increased questioning or information-seeking about the perioperative experience.
- Listen for voice tremors or pitch changes in the patient.
- Listen for increased verbalization by the patient.
- Listen for increased rate of verbalization by the patient.
- Look for hand tremors.
- Determine whether the patient is experiencing increased muscle tension.
- Determine whether the patient has a narrowing focus of attention progressing to a fixed focus.

Assessing Anticipatory Anxiety in the Patient (Gordon, 1987a, pp. 200, 202)

- Listen for verbalization of apprehension, uncertainty, fear, distress, or worry.
- Listen for verbalization of painful and persistent feelings of increased helplessness, inadequacy, regret.
- Look for expressions of concern (change in life events).
- Look for signs of fear of unspecified consequences.
- Look for signs that the patient is overexcited, rattled, jittery, or scared.
- Determine whether the patient shows restlessness, focus on self, insomnia, increased perspiration.
- Watch the patient for signs of increased wariness, glancing about, poor eye contact, facial tension, voice quivering.
- Look for increased tension, foot shuffling, hand/arm movements, trembling, hand tremor, shakiness.

Assessing the Presence of Body Image Disturbance

- Determine whether surgery will entail removal of a body part significant to sexual identity.
- Determine whether surgery will result in a change in the appearance of body parts visible to others (face, neck, hands).
- Determine whether surgery will result in amputation of a limb.

- Listen for verbalization by the patient that he or she will experience difficulty in integrating the impending body change.
- Listen for verbalization by the patient that the body will be imperfect after surgery.

Assessing the Presence of Anticipatory Grieving
(Gordon, 1987a, p. 228)

- Listen for verbal expression of distress at potential (anticipated) loss.
- Look for signs of anger.
- Watch for signs of sadness, sorrow, crying.
- Determine whether the patient cries at frequent intervals or has a choked feeling.
- Determine whether the patient has had a change in eating habits.
- Assess the patient's sleep or dream patterns.
- Determine whether the patient has experienced changes in activity level.
- Determine whether the patient has had changes in libido.
- Assess whether the patient has idealized the anticipated loss.
- Look for signs of developmental regression.
- Assess whether the patient has experienced alterations in concentration or pursuit of tasks.

Assessing the Patient's Ability to Cope (Gordon, 1987a, p. 284)

- Listen for verbalization of inability to cope.
- Determine whether the patient is able to ask for help.
- Assess whether the patient is able to effectively solve problems.
- Determine whether the patient is experiencing anxiety, fear, anger, irritability, tension.
- Determine the presence of life stress (such as a major surgical experience or disease process).
- Ask if the patient is able to meet role expectations (such as a permanent or temporary loss of employment as a consequence of surgery).
- Determine whether the patient is able to meet basic needs.
- Look for clues of the patient's ability to participate in societal activities.
- Determine whether the patient has demonstrated destructive behavior toward self and others.
- Assess whether the patient uses appropriate and effective defense mechanisms.
- Determine whether the patient has experienced a change in usual communication patterns.

- Ask if the patient has had an excess in food intake, alcohol consumption, or smoking.
- Determine whether the patient has had a change in digestive ability, bowel habits, appetite.
- Ask if the patient is experiencing chronic fatigue or sleep pattern disturbance.

Assessing the Family's Ability to Cope (Gordon, 1987a, p. 300)

- Determine whether the family has neglected caring for the patient with regard to basic human needs or treatment of illness.
- Determine whether the family has a distorted view of reality concerning the patient's health problem or denial of the existence or the severity of the disease process.
- Look for signs of family intolerance toward the patient.
- Assess whether the family has rejected, abandoned, or deserted the patient.
- Look for behaviors that indicate that the family is carrying on usual routines while disregarding the patient's needs.
- Watch for clues of the family's taking on illness signs of the patient.
- Determine whether the patient is implementing decisions and actions that are detrimental to his or her economic or social well-being.
- Watch for family demonstration of agitation, aggression, or hostility toward the patient.
- Determine whether family members are experiencing depression.
- Look for signs of neglectful relationship with other family members.
- Determine whether the patient demonstrates helpless or inactive dependence behaviors.

PATIENT OUTCOME STANDARDS

This section identifies patient outcome standards for the critical competencies of perioperative nursing practice as identified by the Association of Operating Room Nurses, Inc., AORN (1993), and the authors:

- Preparing the patient for surgery
- Transferring the patient
- Patient and family teaching
- Performing sponge, sharps, and instrument counts
- Providing instruments, equipment, and supplies
- Administering drugs and solutions
- Physiologically monitoring the patient
- Monitoring and controlling the environment
- Positioning the patient
- Handling cultures and specimens
- Handling tissues with instruments
- Providing hemostasis
- Facilitating postoperative care

The standards will assist the perioperative nurse or the registered nurse first assistant (RNFA) in identifying critical perioperative nursing diagnoses and defining expected outcomes for the surgical patient.

PREPARING THE PATIENT FOR SURGERY
Standard

The patient receives care that reflects an ongoing process of management of his or her health status during the perioperative period.

Criteria

Depending on the patient's physical, psychological, sociocultural, and spiritual status, the patient or the significant other (if applicable) can expect a plan of care that ensures that the patient

- Complies with the prescribed therapeutic regimen before and after surgery

- Is free from nosocomial infection after surgery
- Is free from injury related to electrical and radiation hazards, chemicals, extraneous objects, positioning, the administration of drugs and solutions, the improper handling of culture and specimens, and the handling of tissue with instruments during surgery
- Maintains fluid volume
- Maintains skin and tissue integrity
- Maintains body temperature within normal limits
- Is free from prolonged adynamic ileus following surgery
- Demonstrates self-care activities after surgery
- Demonstrates effective airway clearance
- Demonstrates effective postoperative breathing patterns
- Maintains cardiac output
- Has adequate postoperative tissue perfusion
- Experiences minimal postoperative pain
- Is knowledgeable about the perioperative experience
- Copes with feelings of fear before surgery
- Recognizes the presence of anticipatory anxiety
- Copes with changes in body image after surgery
- Recognizes the presence of anticipatory grief and demonstrates function grieving
- Demonstrates effective coping in response to the stress of impending surgery

TRANSFERRING THE PATIENT
Standard

Preoperative and postoperative transfer activities do not compromise or cause injury to the patient.

Criteria

The patient is free from evidence of
- Tissue injury
- Altered body temperature
- Ineffective breathing patterns
- Altered tissue perfusion
- Discomfort or pain
- Fear

PATIENT AND FAMILY TEACHING
Standard

The patient and/or family members demonstrate knowledge concerning surgical intervention.

Criteria

The patient and/or family members demonstrate knowledge of
- Perioperative environment and pertinent aspects of the surgical procedure
- Potential physical and psychological effects of surgery
- Coping mechanisms that can be used in response to surgical intervention
- How to participate in the rehabilitation process after surgery

CREATING AND MAINTAINING A STERILE FIELD
Standard

Creating and maintaining a sterile field do not compromise or cause injury to the patient.

Criteria

The patient is free from evidence of
- Postoperative wound infection
- Impaired skin integrity
- Hyperthermia
- Hypothermia
- Ineffective breathing patterns
- Disturbed self-esteem

PERFORMING SPONGE, SHARPS, AND INSTRUMENT COUNTS
Standard

The patient is free from injury related to the retention of sponges, sharps, or instruments.

Criteria

There is an absence of
- Unexplained pain, cramping, and fever
- Formation of abscesses in the abdominal, retroperitoneal, and chest cavities
- Images of retained sponges, sharps, or instruments on the patient's x-ray films

PROVIDING INSTRUMENTS, EQUIPMENT, AND SUPPLIES
Standard

The patient is free from injury related to the provision of instruments, equipment, and supplies during surgery.

Criteria

The patient is free from evidence of
- Alterations in temperature
- Electrical injury
- Burns
- Nosocomial infection

ADMINISTERING DRUGS AND SOLUTIONS
Standard

The patient is free from injury related to the administration of medications and solutions.

Criteria

The patient is free from injury during the intraoperative phase and any sequela during the postoperative phase. There are no signs of
- Drug overdose
- Drug toxicity
- Allergic reactions

PHYSIOLOGICALLY MONITORING THE PATIENT
Standard I

The patient's breathing patterns are maintained during surgery.

Criteria

Depending on the physical and psychological status, the patient exhibits no signs of
- Ineffective airway clearance
- Respiratory depression related to IV sedation

Standard II

The patient is free from injuries associated with IV fluid intake.

Criteria

Depending on the physical and psychological status, the patient exhibits no signs of
- Alteration in cardiac output related to air embolism associated with fluid administration
- Alteration in tissue integrity related to infiltration of IV fluid
- Alteration in fluid volume related to the administration of excessive fluid

Standard III

The patient maintains a balanced circulating blood volume.

Criteria

Depending on the physical and psychological status, the patient exhibits no signs of fluid deficit associated with intraoperative blood loss.

Standard IV

The patient maintains normal body temperature.

Criteria

Depending on the physical and psychological status, the patient exhibits no signs of hypothermia or hyperthermia.

Standard V

The patient is free from complications associated with the administration of local anesthesia.

Criteria

Depending on the physical and psychological status, the patient exhibits no signs of

- Impaired tissue integrity related to extravasation of medication
- Allergic reaction to the local anesthetic
- Toxic effects of the local anesthetic

MONITORING AND CONTROLLING THE ENVIRONMENT
Standard

The patient is free from injury related to environmental hazards.

Criteria

The patient is free from evidence of
- Alterations in temperature
- Electrical injury
- Radiation injury
- Nosocomial infection
- Fear

POSITIONING THE PATIENT
Standard

Surgical positioning does not physiologically compromise or cause injury to the patient.

Criteria

There are no signs or symptoms of
- Physical injury reported by the patient or significant others

- Impaired skin integrity or breakdown
- Ineffective breathing
- Altered tissue perfusion
- Postoperative pain
- Uncompensated deficit (touch or kinesthesia)

HANDLING CULTURES AND SPECIMENS
Standard

The patient is free from injury related to the handling of cultures and specimens during the perioperative period.

Criteria

The patient does not experience a compromised diagnosis because of inappropriate handling of cultures and specimens.

HANDLING TISSUE WITH INSTRUMENTS
Standard

Handling tissue with instruments does not compromise or cause injury to the patient.

Criteria

The patient is free from evidence of
- Postoperative hematoma
- Serous discharge or local infection
- Wound dehiscence
- Excessive scar formation
- Postoperative neuromuscular impairment
- Postoperative impaired tissue integrity

PROVIDING HEMOSTASIS
Standard

Providing hemostasis does not compromise or cause injury to the patient.

Criteria

Depending on the patient's health status, the patient is free from evidence of
- Postoperative infection related to the use of intraoperative thermal and chemical hemostatic techniques
- Injury related to the use of intraoperative mechanical, chemical, and thermal hemostatic techniques
- Intraoperative or postoperative fluid volume deficit

FACILITATING POSTOPERATIVE CARE
Standard I

The patient experiences uncomplicated wound healing.

Criteria

The wound appears
- Pink (free from tissue necrosis and inflammation)
- Flat (free from hematoma or serum fluid collection)
- Intact (with skin edges sealed)
- Dry (free from purulent or serous drainage)
- Soft (free from spreading induration)

Standard II

The patient remains free from wound infection after surgery.

Criteria

The patient is free from
- Chills and fever
- Redness, warmth, and swelling around the incision or open wounds
- Unusual drainage from wound
- White blood cell count beyond normal limits

Standard III

The patient is free from systemic postoperative complications.

Criteria

The following demonstrate freedom from systemic complications
- Oral temperature below 100°F
- Normal urine output (about 30 ml/hour or greater)
- Absence of frequency or burning on urination
- Return of bowel sounds and function in an appropriate amount of time
- Normal breath sounds and respiratory rate
- Heart rate within normal limits
- Absence of pain and swelling in the extremities

Standard IV

The patient experiences physiologic and psychological comfort after surgery.

Criteria

The following demonstrates an acceptable comfort level
- Absence of nausea, vomiting, and hiccups

- Verbalization of adequate pain relief
- Relaxed facial expression
- Gradual increase in activity level

PERIOPERATIVE NURSING DIAGNOSES

The perioperative nursing diagnoses listed in this section are categorized according to functional health patterns. This is not an all-inclusive list. Rather, the list demonstrates the many types of diagnosis that may be seen in the surgical patient.

HEALTH PERCEPTION–HEALTH MANAGEMENT PATTERN
Diagnosis

High risk for infection.

Definition

Presence of risk factors for the patient to experience a nosocomial infection secondary to exposure to the surgical environment.

Risk Factors (Gordon, 1987a, p. 50)

- Surgical intervention that alters tissue and skin integrity
- Inadequate secondary defenses (e.g., decreased hemoglobin concentration, leukopenia, suppressed inflammatory response, and immunosuppression)
- Inadequate acquired immunity (e.g., acquired immunodeficiency syndrome)
- Chronic disease leading to suppressed immunity (e.g., lupus erythematosus)
- Altered tissue perfusion
- Invasive drains and monitors (intravenous catheters, hyperalimentation catheters, nasogastric tubes, Foley catheters, chest tubes)
- Malnutrition that interferes with tissue repair
- Blood abnormalities such as sickle cell anemia, thrombocytopenia, and thalassemia
- Impaired skin integrity
- Impaired tissue integrity
- Failure of sterilization or disinfection processes

- Nonadherence to surgical suite traffic patterns
- Failure of environmental sanitation processes
- Existing acquired infection
- Increased environmental exposure due to the length of surgery
- Break in aseptic technique
- Improper wearing of surgical attire resulting in shedding or spraying of microorganisms from the surgical team into the sterile field
- Extremes of age
- Type of procedure that predisposes to possible infection (gastrointestinal and genitourinary tract surgery, surgery on injured or ischemic tissue, denuded bone, implanted foreign bodies or prosthetic devices)

Expected Outcome

The patient is free from nosocomial infection after surgery.
- Does the patient show evidence of wound infection?
- Does the patient have a urinary tract infection?
- Does the patient have an upper respiratory tract infection?

The patient is free from wound infection 72 hours postoperatively.
- Does the patient complain of chills or fever?
- Is there redness, warmth, and swelling around the incision or open wounds?
- Is there an unusual amount of wound drainage?
- Is the white blood cell count within normal limits?
- Are there positive cultures of wound drainage?
- Is cellulitis present?
- Are there signs and symptoms of an abscess?
- Does the patient have lymphangitis?
- Are there signs and symptoms of gas gangrene?
- Are there signs and symptoms of Meleney's ulcer?
- Did the patient experience wound dehiscence? (Rothrock, 1987, pp. 191–192)

Diagnosis

High risk for infection related to the use of microfibrillar collagen hemostat, gelatin sponge, and oxidized cellulose.

Definition

Presence of risk factors for the patient to experience postoperative infection related to the use of microfibrillar collagen hemostat, gelatin sponge, and oxidized cellulose to achieve hemostasis.

MICROFIBRILLAR COLLAGEN HEMOSTAT
- Suppressed immune system secondary to blood transfusions
- Retained blood products in the subcutaneous tissue (retained blood products provide an excellent growth medium for bacteria)

GELATIN SPONGE
- Allergy to gelatin products
- Inflammation of the operative site, wound contamination, or infection
- Application of product to wound edges

OXIDIZED CELLULOSE
- Contaminated wound
- Suppressed immune system secondary to blood transfusions
- Retained blood products in the subcutaneous tissue

Expected Outcome

The patient is free from postoperative infection related to the use of microfibrillar collagen hemostat, gelatin sponge, and oxidized cellulose to achieve intraoperative hemostasis.
- Does the patient complain of chills and fever?
- Is the wound red, warm to touch, and swollen?
- Is there an unusual amount of wound drainage?
- Is the white blood cell count within normal limits?
- Are there positive cultures from wound drainage?

Diagnosis

High risk for infection related to wound dehiscence or evisceration.

Definition

Presence of risk factors for the patient to experience wound infection and peritonitis related to wound dehiscence and evisceration after surgery.

Risk Factors

- Inadequate wound closure
- Wounds closed under tension
- Compromised wound healing

Expected Outcome

The patient is free from wound infection and peritonitis.
- Does the patient demonstrate evidence of wound infection?
- Does the patient show evidence of peritonitis?

Diagnosis

High risk for infection related to seroma formation in the postoperative wound.

Definition

Presence of risk factors for the patient to experience a postoperative wound infection after the formation of a seroma.

Risk Factors
- Obesity
- Surgical wound with areas of undermined skin flaps

Expected Outcome
The patient is free from postoperative wound infection related to seroma formation.
- Does the patient complain of chills and fever?
- Is there redness, warmth, and swelling around the incision or open wounds?
- Is there an unusual amount of wound drainage?
- Is there an abnormal white blood cell count and positive cultures of wound drainage?

Diagnosis
High risk for postoperative urinary tract infection.

Definition
Presence of risk factors for the patient to experience a urinary tract infection after surgery.

Risk Factors
- Dehydration
- Urinary retention
- Indwelling urinary catheter

Expected Outcome
The patient remains free from a urinary tract infection.
- Is the patient's urine clear?
- Is there an unusual odor to the patient's urine?
- Does the patient complain of urinary frequency, urgency, or burning on urination?
- Is there an absence of chills or fever?
- Are white blood cells or bacteria present in the urine?
- Does the patient have a positive or negative urine culture?

Diagnosis
High risk for injury related to transfer to and from the surgical suite.

Definition
Presence of risk factors that may cause the patient to experience bodily injury while being transported to and from the surgical suite and during transfer activities.

Risk Factors

- Neuromuscular impairment
- Musculoskeletal impairment
- Vascular impairment
- Cognitive impairment
- Sensory/perceptual impairment (vision, hearing)
- Speech impairment
- Safety violations by the transporter
- Equipment malfunction
- Extraneous objects (hanging intravenous [IV] bags, patient drainage devices)

Expected Outcome

The patient shows no subjective or objective evidence of injury.

- Does the patient or family verbally or nonverbally complain of injury?
- Are there signs of broken or bruised skin?

Diagnosis

High risk for injury related to retained sponges, sharps, and instruments.

Definition

Presence of risk factors for the patient to experience injury because of sponges, sharps, or instruments inadvertently left in the surgical wound after closure.

Risk Factors

- Emergency surgery that precludes counting of sponges, sharps, and instruments
- Intraoperative hemorrhaging necessitating the immediate use of a great number of sponges
- Surgery entailing the packing of cavities with sponges
- Change of perioperative nursing staff during the procedure
- Lenient institutional count policies and procedures
- Use of small instruments in deep cavities

Expected Outcome

The patient does not exhibit signs or symptoms indicating the retention of sponges, sharps, or instruments after surgery.

- Does the patient have signs and symptoms of fever?
- Does the patient complain of pain unrelated to incisional pain?
- Are there signs of intestinal obstruction?
- Are there signs of abscess formation?

Diagnosis

High risk for injury related to the use of electrocautery to achieve hemostasis.

Definition

Presence of risk factors for the patient to experience skin damage, hemorrhage, hematoma formation, postoperative pain, and neurologic deficit related to the use of electrocautery to achieve intraoperative hemostasis.

Risk Factors (Association of Operating Room Nurses [AORN], 1993, pp. 121–123, 138–139)

- Excessive hair at dispersive electrode site
- Scar tissue at dispersive electrode site
- Internal or external metal prosthetic devices at the dispersive electrode site
- Impaired skin or tissue integrity, bony prominences, or impaired tissue perfusion at site of dispersive electrode or electrocardiographic lead placement
- Pacemakers
- Frayed or damaged power cords
- Damaged outlets
- Malfunctioning isolated power system
- Improper application of dispersive electrode
- Use of faulty equipment
- Use of inflammable agents to prepare the operative site
- Obesity (excessive subcutaneous tissue does not conduct electricity well)
- Use of rectal probes
- Exposed metal touching the patient's skin
- Defective electrosurgical dispersive pad
- Tension on the active and dispersive electrode cords

Expected Outcome

The patient is free from injury related to the application of electrocautery to achieve intraoperative hemostasis.

- Does the patient show evidence of impaired skin and tissue integrity at dispersive electrode and electrocardiographic lead sites?
- Was there evidence of intraoperative hemorrhage?
- Does the patient show evidence of postoperative impaired tissue integrity (hematoma formation) and deep tissue burns?
- Does the patient complain of postoperative pain or neurologic deficit surrounding the cautery site?
- Does the patient show evidence of impaired skin and tissue integrity at sites where the patient may have contacted metal?

- Is there evidence of altered tissue perfusion?
- Did the patient experience altered cardiac output during the use of electrical equipment?

Diagnosis

High risk for injury related to the use of a pneumatic tourniquet.

Definition

Presence of risk factors for the patient to experience impaired skin and tissue integrity, chemical skin burns, and nerve damage secondary to improper pneumatic tourniquet use.

Risk Factors (AORN, 1993, pp. 169–171)

- Improper cuff size
- Wrinkled padding
- Improper cuff positioning
- Cuff rotation after application
- Pooling of preparation solutions under the cuff
- Excessive cuff pressure
- Excessive cuff inflation time

Expected Outcome (AORN, 1993, pp. 169–171)

The patient is free from injury related to pneumatic tourniquet use.

- Does the patient show evidence of skin bruising, blistering, pinching, or necrosis?
- Does the patient have skin abrasions or swelling at the tourniquet site?
- Is the tourniquet site free from evidence of chemical skin burns?
- Are there signs of paralysis or other signs of nerve damage in the extremity of tourniquet application?

Diagnosis

High risk for injury related to hypersensitivity reaction because of improper identification of patient allergies.

Definition

Presence of risk factors for the patient to experience a hypersensitivity reaction during drug administration owing to unidentified allergies.

Risk Factors

- History of a past reaction to specific or related anti-infective agents
- History of self-treatment with anti-infective drugs

- Inability of the patient or family members to provide an accurate drug history
- Use of anti-infective drugs for self-treatment of minor infections

Expected Outcome

The patient undergoes the surgical procedure without evidence or report of local or systemic drug reaction.

- Is the patient uneasy, apprehensive, and weak?
- Does the patient express a feeling of impending doom?
- Does the patient demonstrate generalized pruritus and urticaria?
- Does the patient have erythema and angioedema of the eyes, lips, or tongue?
- Are discrete cutaneous wheals or urticarial eruptions present?
- Does the patient have congestion, rhinorrhea, dyspnea, and increasing respiratory distress with audible wheezing?
- Are rales, wheezing, and diminished breath sounds present?
- Is there hypotension and a rapid, weak pulse?
- Does the patient complain of abdominal cramping, diarrhea, or vomiting? (Ignatavicius and Bayne, 1991, p. 654)

Diagnosis

High risk for injury related to hypersensitivity or an adverse reaction to an anticoagulant.

Definition

Presence of risk factors for the patient to experience an allergic reaction to the administration of anticoagulants.

Risk Factors

- History of allergic hypersensitivity to heparin, dextran 40 injection, or other anticoagulant
- Heparin resistance resulting from large amounts of fibrin deposits in conditions such as early-stage thrombophlebitis, peritonitis, fever, pleurisy, cancer, myocardial infarction, and extensive surgery
- Dextran sensitivity (a small percentage of persons who never received dextran experience an allergic reaction because of previous sensitization by the dextrans present in commercial sugars and dextran-producing organisms found in the human gastrointestinal tract)

Expected Outcome

The patient is free from an allergic reaction to anticoagulant therapy.

- Does the patient complain of chills?

- Does the patient have a fever?
- Does the patient have a rash, urticaria?
- Are anaphylactic and anaphylactoid reactions present?.

Diagnosis

High risk for injury related to the administration of a local anesthetic.

Definition

Presence of risk factors for the patient's experiencing an allergic reaction to a local anesthetic agent.

Risk Factors

- Sensitivity to local anesthetic, methylparaben, or p-aminobenzoic acid (PABA)
- Patients with hepatic dysfunction, congestive heart failure, and cardiogenic shock (these patients tend to metabolize local anesthetic drugs at a slower rate than usual)
- Patients at risk for malignant hyperthermia

Expected Outcome

The patient is free from allergic reaction related to the administration local anesthetic agents.

- Does the patient manifest allergic responses such as redness, rash, urticaria, and bronchoconstriction?

Diagnosis

High risk for injury related to toxicity of a local anesthetic.

Definition

Presence of risk factors for the patient to experience a toxic reaction to a local anesthetic agent.

Risk Factors

- Systemic diseases that slow the metabolism of the local anesthetic agent (a pseudocholinesterase deficiency increases the chance of toxic responses with an amino ester agent)

Expected Outcome

The patient is free from allergic or toxic reaction related to the administration of local anesthetic agents.

- Is the patient apprehensive?
- Does the patient have blurred vision, tinnitus, or dizziness?
- Is the patient awake and alert?
- Are there signs of central nervous system depression or respiratory depression?

Diagnosis

High risk for injury related to mydriatic agent administration causing an acute angle-closure glaucoma episode.

Definition

Presence of risk factors for the patient to experience an acute glaucoma episode owing to the inadvertent administration of a mydriatic agent.

Risk Factors

- History of angle-closure glaucoma
- Age 40 years or older

Expected Outcome

The patient undergoes an eye examination or ophthalmologic surgery without experiencing an episode of acute angle-closure glaucoma.

- Did the patient experience an episode of acute angle-closure glaucoma?

Diagnosis

High risk for injury related to an allergic or adverse reaction because of patient sensitivity to otic medications.

Definition

Presence of risk factors for the patient to experience injury as a result of the allergic response or other adverse reaction to the administration of an otic preparation.

Risk Factors

- Hypersensitivity to any of the components of antibiotics
- Presence of secondary infections in chronic dermatoses

Expected Outcome

The patient receives otic suspensions or solutions without an allergic or adverse reaction.

- Does the patient complain of pruritus?
- Is swelling or inflammation evident?
- Are there other clinical manifestations of allergic reaction or secondary infection?

Diagnosis

High risk for injury related to an allergic reaction to contrast media.

Definition

Presence of risk factors for the patient to experience an allergic reaction to contrast media during a radiographic examination.

Risk Factors

- History of allergy to contrast media or a related compound.
- Hypersensitivity to iodine
- Bronchial asthma
- Hay fever
- Food allergies, such as shellfish allergy

Expected Outcome

The patient does not experience injury (allergic reaction) related to the administration of contrast media.

- Does the patient manifest respiratory, central nervous system, cardiovascular, renal, or local reactions?

Diagnosis

High risk for injury related to devices used to assist patient recovery.

Definition

Presence of risk factors for the patient to experience bodily injury (i.e., impaired skin integrity, damage to internal organs) from devices used to assist during recovery.

Risk Factors

Malfunctioning or improperly applied:

- Nasogastric tube
- Taped pressure dressing
- Chest tubes
- Closed-wound drainage devices
- Open-wound drainage devices

Expected Outcome

The patient remains injury free.

- Are there signs of impaired skin integrity?
- Are there signs of damage to internal organs?

Diagnosis

High risk for injury related to ionizing radiation exposure.

Definition

Presence of risk factors for the patient to experience injury from exposure to ionizing radiation.

Risk Factors
- Fluoroscopy
- Multiple x-ray films during surgery
- Pregnancy

Expected Outcome
The patient is free from injury related to ionizing radiation.
- If the patient is pregnant, was the fetus exposed to radiation?
- Are there signs of tissue trauma (burns)?
- Does the patient show evidence of anemia following radiation exposure?
- Does the patient show evidence of sterility following radiation exposure?

Diagnosis

High risk for injury related to nonionizing radiation exposure.

Definition
Presence of risk factors for the patient to experience impaired skin and tissue integrity from exposure to laser beams.

Risk Factors
- Unprotected eyes during laser use
- Aberrant and reflected laser beams
- Plume and noxious fumes
- Use of flammable or combustible anesthetics, preparation solutions, drying agents, ointments, plastic resins, or plastics

Diagnosis

High risk for injury related to surgical positioning.

Definition
Presence of risk factors for the patient to experience bodily injury because of surgical positioning.

Risk Factors
- Disorientation
- Impaired judgment
- Paralysis/neuromuscular impairment
- Musculoskeletal impairment
- Sensory/perceptual deterioration due to disease, medication, or anesthesia
- Existing or previous trauma or accidental injury

- Lack of safety precautions attributed to inadequate, untrained, or inattentive staff, a shortage of equipment, and a hazardous environment
- Presence of internal or external prosthetic devices

Expected Outcome

The patient is free from injury related to nonionizing radiation.
- Does the patient show evidence of retinal trauma?
- Does the patient show evidence of impaired tissue or skin integrity?
- Does the patient demonstrate respiratory difficulty related to breathing laser plume or noxious odors?

Diagnosis

High risk for injury related to improper handling of cultures and specimens obtained during surgery.

Definition

Presence of risk factors for the patient to experience a wrong diagnosis, no diagnosis, or the prevention of definitive therapy because of improper handling of cultures and specimens by the perioperative nursing team.

Risk Factors

- Failure to provide the correct supplies and equipment for culture and specimen collection
- Incorrect labeling of culture and tissue specimen containers
- Incorrect completion of laboratory slips
- Incorrect documentation of cultures and specimens on the patient's operative record
- Failure to establish chain of custody for cultures and tissue specimens
- Improper intraoperative processing of cultures and tissue for examination
- Improper storage, preservation, and maintenance of tissue
- Failure to properly direct the transfer of cultures and specimens to the laboratory
- Incorrect communication of intraoperative pathology reports to the surgeon

Expected Outcome

The patient is free from injury related to the handling of specimens and cultures.
- Is there evidence of incorrect medical diagnosis?

- Is there evidence of incorrect treatment due to improper handling of cultures and specimens by the perioperative nursing team?

Diagnosis

High risk for injury related to handling of tissue with instruments during surgery.

Definition

Presence of risk factors for the patient to experience postoperative impaired physical mobility, impaired tissue integrity, altered tissue perfusion, and discomfort related to the exposure, clamping, grasping, suturing, and cutting of tissue during surgery.

Risk Factors (Rothrock, 1987, pp. 124–125; Ethicon, 1988, p. 5)

- Altered circulation
- Obesity
- Emaciation
- Extremes in age, height, and body build
- Presence of physical deformities or limitations
- Failure to evaluate the type of tissue, location of vascular or nerve structures, and the presence of organs in relation to the method used to provide exposure
- Inadequate hemostasis
- Extended surgical procedure
- Excessive intraoperative abduction or adduction of extremities
- Direct pressure on body surface from members of the surgical team
- Exposure of the operative site with a retractor intended for use only on selected surgical procedures or on a specific type of tissue
- Use of an intestinal bag
- Excessive or improper retraction of tissue
- Improper clamping or grasping of tissue

Expected Outcome

The patient is free from injury related to the handling of tissue with instruments.

- Does the patient show evidence of impaired physical mobility (inability to move, decreased active joint range of motion, and decreased muscle strength or control) after surgery?
- Does the patient show evidence of impaired tissue integrity (excessive swelling at the surgical site, skin discoloration on body surfaces) after surgery?

- Does the patient show evidence of altered tissue perfusion (cold extremities, diminished arterial pulses, blood pressure changes in extremities, discoloration of an extremity) after surgery? (Gordon, 1987a, p. 160)
- Does the patient complain of excessive discomfort (excluding incisional pain) after surgery?

Diagnosis

High risk for injury related to the use of a laser to achieve hemostasis.

Definition

Presence of risk factors for the patient to experience skin damage around the operative site and corneal burns related to the use of a laser to achieve intraoperative hemostasis.

Risk Factors (AORN, 1993, pp. 155–157)

- Movement during laser operation
- Use of inflammable draping material
- Poor exposure of the operative field
- Use of reflective instruments
- Use of dry sponges during laser operation
- Inadequate eye protection for the patient
- Use of nonlaser endotracheal tube
- Exposed tissue around the operative field

Expected Outcome

The patient is free from injury related to the use of laser equipment to achieve intraoperative hemostasis.

- Is there evidence of impaired tissue integrity surrounding the operative site?
- Does patient show evidence of corneal burns?

Diagnosis

High risk for injury related to the use of mechanical methods to achieve hemostasis.

Definition

Presence of risk factors for the patient to experience injury related to the use of pressure and the application of hemostatic clips to achieve intraoperative hemostasis.

Risk Factors

- Adhesions

- Obesity (excessive tissue mass impedes exposure of the operative field, which may interfere with the use of pressure or the application of hemostatic clips)
- Poor operative exposure
- Use of packs to stop bleeding
- Application of inappropriate-sized clip
- Defective clip appliers
- Improper identification of anatomic structure before clipping

Expected Outcome

The patient is free from injury related to the use of mechanical methods to achieve hemostasis.

- Does the patient show evidence of intraoperative fluid deficit such as hemorrhage due to the improper use of pressure or application of hemostatic clips?
- Does the patient show evidence of postoperative infection or pain related to retained packing sponges?
- Does the patient show evidence of postoperative pain or neurologic deficit related to inadvertent clipping of nerves surrounding the bleeding site?
- Does the patient have impaired tissue integrity such as damaged or destroyed integumentary and subcutaneous tissue related to inadvertent use of excessive pressure or clipping of tissue surrounding the bleeding site?

Diagnosis

High risk for injury related to the use of microfibrillar collagen hemostat.

Definition

The presence of risk factors for the patient to experience abscess and hematoma formation, bone and tissue injury due to insecure orthopedic prosthesis, nonhealing of wound skin edges, bowel adhesion, compromised urinary output, aspiration, blood contamination, and allergic response related to the use of microfibrillar collagen hemostat to achieve intraoperative hemostasis.

Risk Factors

- Use of methylmethacrylate (agent significantly reduces the bonding strength of methylmethacrylate)
- Application to wound edges
- Failure to remove excess amounts of agent
- Use of blood scavaging systems
- Allergy to bovine products

Expected Outcome

The patient is free from injury related to the use of microfibrillar collagen hemostat to achieve intraoperative hemostasis.

- Is there evidence of abscess or hematoma formation?
- Is there evidence of failure of orthopedic prosthesis due to a reduction of bonding strength of methylmethacrylate?
- Is there evidence of nonhealing of wound skin edges?
- Does the patient show evidence of bowel adhesion?
- Does the patient show evidence of compromised urinary output due to mechanical pressure against the ureter?
- Is there evidence of aspiration of microfibrillar collagen hemostat?
- Is there evidence of blood contamination with microfibrillar collagen hemostat particles?
- Does the patient show evidence of allergic response to microfibrillar collagen hemostat?

Diagnosis

High risk for injury related to the use of collagen sponge.

Definition

Presence of risk factors for the patient to experience hematoma formation, pain, and neurologic deficit related to the use of collagen sponge to achieve intraoperative hemostasis.

Risk Factors

- Allergy to materials of bovine origin
- Use in urologic, ophthalmologic, and neurologic replacement procedures
- Use in the presence of methylmethacrylate
- Application to wound edges

Expected Outcome

The patient is free from injury related to the use of collagen sponge to achieve intraoperative hemostasis.

- Is there evidence of hematoma formation due to vascular oozing from improper application or use of gelatin sponge?
- Does the patient complain of pain/discomfort suggesting formation of adhesions?
- Are there signs of allergic reaction to collagen sponge?
- Is there evidence of postoperative pain or neurologic deficit related to the application of collagen sponge?

Diagnosis

High risk for injury related to the use of oxidized cellulose for hemostasis.

Definition

Presence of risk factors for the patient to experience interference with callus formation in bone defects, stenosis of vascular structures, headaches, sneezing, and burning and stinging sensations to localized application areas related to the use of collagen sponge to achieve intraoperative hemostasis.

Risk Factors

- Orthopedic surgery
- Spinal cord and optic nerve surgery
- Vascular surgery
- Nasal surgery (polypectomy) when oxidized cellulose is used for packing
- Hemorrhoidectomy, skin graft donor sites, and dermabrasion

Expected Outcome

The patient is free from injury related to the use of oxidized cellulose for hemostasis.

- Are there signs of impaired bone healing?
- Are there signs of vascular stenosis?
- Does the patient complain of headaches?
- Does the patient complain of sneezing or of burning and stinging sensations to localized application areas?

Diagnosis

High risk for noncompliance with the prescribed therapeutic regimen after surgery.

Definition

Presence of risk factors for the patient's or family members' nonadherence to the prescribed postoperative treatment regimen.

Risk Factors (Gordon, 1987a, p. 48)

- History of noncompliance with aspects of therapeutic regimen
- Lack of support systems (family, friends)
- Denial of illness
- Perceived ineffectiveness of recommended treatment
- Perceived lack of seriousness of problems or risk factors
- Perceived lack of suspectibility
- Insufficient knowledge or skills

- Absence of a plan for integrating therapeutic recommendations into daily routines

Expected Outcome

The patient complies with the prescribed therapeutic regimen after surgery.

- Is the patient noncompliant with therapeutic regimen observed by the nurse?
- Does the patient or significant other make statements describing noncompliance?
- Do objective tests (such as physiologic measures) reveal noncompliance?
- Is there evidence of the development of complications?
- Is there evidence of exacerbation of symptoms?
- Does the patient fail to keep appointments?
- Does the patient fail to progress or resolve an identified problem? (Gordon, 1987a, p. 48)

NUTRITIONAL-METABOLIC PATTERN
Diagnosis

High risk for altered body temperature related to transfer to and from the surgical suite.

Definition

Presence of risk factors that may cause the patient to experience a decrease in body temperature (hypothermia) during preoperative and postoperative transfer activities.

Risk Factors (Gordon, 1987a, p. 92)

- Extremes in age (neonate, elderly)
- Extremes in weight
- Fluid deficit (dehydration)
- Altered metabolic rate
- Impaired temperature regulation secondary to illness or injury
- Vasoconstriction or vasodilation secondary to medication
- Cold environmental temperature
- Inadequate covering

Expected Outcome

The patient shows no subjective or objective evidence of a decrease in body temperature during preoperative and postoperative transfer.

- Are there verbal or nonverbal statements (shivering or chattering teeth) of discomfort indicating a decrease in body temperature?

Diagnosis

High risk for hyperthermia during the surgical procedure.

Definition

Presence of risk factors for the patient to experience an elevated body temperature during the intraoperative period.

Risk Factors (Gordon, 1987a, p. 96)

- Existing hyperthermia (fever)
- Patient illness or trauma
- Dehydration
- Low tolerance for heat-retaining devices (blankets)
- Decreased ability to perspire
- Ineffective air-conditioning system in the operating room
- Overapplication of sterile plastic drapes

Expected Outcome

The patient's body temperature is maintained within normal limits during the intraoperative period.

- Did the patient experience an increase in intraoperative body temperature above the normal range?
- Was the patient's skin flushed during the intraoperative period?
- Did the patient have an increase in intraoperative respiratory rate (particularly the nonventilated patient)?
- Was there evidence of intraoperative tachycardia?
- Did the patient have an intraoperative seizure or convulsion? (Gordon, 1987a, p. 96)

Diagnosis

High risk for hypothermia.

Definition

Presence of risk factors for the patient to experience a decreased body temperature during the intraoperative period.

Risk Factors (Gordon, 1987a, p. 98)

- Existing hypothermia
- Impaired skin integrity (i.e., burn patient)
- Low body weight (malnutrition)
- Age—very young or very old
- Inability to shiver
- Decreased metabolic rate
- Low temperature in the operating room (OR)

- Limited application of covers
- Cold solutions such as intravenous fluids, skin preparation solutions, and wound irrigation solutions
- Medication causing vasodilation

Expected Outcome

The patient maintains a normal body temperature during the perioperative period.

- Does the patient have decrease in body temperature below normal range?
- Does the patient's skin feel cool?
- Does the patient show evidence of mental confusion?
- Does the patient have a decrease in pulse and respiration rates? (Gordon, 1987a, p. 98)

Diagnosis

High risk for postoperative hyperthermia (fever).

Definition

Presence of risk factors for the patient to experience an elevated temperature after surgery.

Risk Factors

- Intraoperative blood administration
- Removal of inflamed tissue during surgery
- Decreased ambulation
- Wound complications
- Intraabdominal abscesses or anastomotic leaks
- Thrombophlebitis

Expected Outcome

The patient is free from postoperative fever.

- Does the patient have an elevated temperature?
- Does the patient feel warm to the touch?
- Does the patient complain of feeling feverish?

Diagnosis

High risk for altered body temperature.

Definition

Presence of risk factors for the patient to experience environment-induced hyperthermia or hypothermia while in the surgical suite.

Risk Factors (AORN, 1993, pp. 136–137; Gordon, 1987a, p. 92)

- General or regional anesthesia
- Excessive sedation, especially in the patient receiving a local anesthetic
- Evaporative or conductive heat loss from prepared skin areas
- Use of unwarmed infusion or irrigating solutions
- Ambient room temperature and humidity
- Surgical exposure of the abdominal or thoracic cavities
- Preexisting medical conditions (e.g., hypothyroid or hyperthyroid problems)
- Extremes in age, particularly infants, small children, and geriatric patients
- Decreased body fat for insulation
- Malnourishment
- Debilitated or chronically ill patients
- Anticipated long operative time
- Intracranial surgery

Expected Outcome

Depending on anesthetic technique and level of consciousness, the patient is free from environment-related alterations in body temperature during the perioperative period.

- Is there evidence of hyperthermia (verbal complaint of feeling uncomfortably warm [for a conscious patient], elevated body temperature, perspiration, tachycardia, warm skin, flushed skin, increased respiratory rate, and seizures or convulsions)?
- Is there evidence of hypothermia (verbal complaint of feeling uncomfortably cold [for a conscious patient], shivering, chattering of teeth, cool skin, and decreased pulse and respiration rate)? (Gordon, 1987a, pp. 98–100)

Diagnosis

High risk for impaired skin integrity related to the administration of skin medications.

Definition

Presence of risk factors for the patient to experience altered skin integrity owing to an allergic response to or contact dermatitis from skin medications.

Risk Factors

- Presence of irritating secretions, blood, pus, or infected drainage

- History of sensitivity to the specific agent or a related compound
- Existing impaired skin integrity

Expected Outcome

The patient's skin remains intact after the application of skin medications.
- Is the patient's skin red after application of skin medication?
- Is swelling present?
- Does the skin have drainage?
- Are there other signs of local irritation?

Diagnosis

High risk for impaired skin integrity related to creation and maintenance of the sterile field.

Definition

Presence of risk factors for skin disruption or breakdown, particularly around the operative site.

Risk Factors (Gordon, 1987a, p. 84)

- Impaired tissue perfusion at the operative site
- Allergy or sensitivity to the prepping solution
- Allergy or sensitivity to an adhesive agent in the draping materials
- Obesity
- Gross underweight
- Poor skin turgor
- Pooling of prepping solutions
- Improper application of towel clips

Expected Outcome

The patient's skin integrity is not impaired by the creation and maintenance of the sterile field.
- Was the patient's skin punctured by towel clips?
- Did adhesive drapes disrupt the patient's skin surface?
- Is there evidence of skin surface breakdown related to pooled prepping solution?

Diagnosis

High risk for impaired skin integrity: nonhealing wound.

Definition

Presence of risk factors for the patient to experience impaired wound healing after surgery.

Risk Factors

- Infection
- Hematomas
- Seromas
- Retained foreign substances
- Underlying disease or conditions
- Alteration in tissue perfusion due to excessive wound tension
- Adjacent tissue scarring or trauma
- Altered circulation to the affected areas due to swelling
- Exudates irritating to the skin
- Use of cytotoxic substances to clean the wound
- Chemical irritation of substances used to clean an open wound
- Obesity
- Use of tape
- Pressure from drain tubes

Expected Outcome

The patient experiences optimal wound healing.
- Are there signs and symptoms of abscess formation?
- Are there signs and symptoms of impending wound dehiscence?
- Are there signs and symptoms of wound infection?
- Does the patient complain of pain beyond what is normal for a healing wound?
- Does the wound have drainage, redness, or swelling?

Diagnosis

High risk for impaired tissue integrity related to the formation of gas gangrene.

Definition

Presence of risk factors for the patient to experience damage to the integumentary or subcutaneous tissue owing to the formation of gas gangrene.

Risk Factors

- Wound contamination with hemolytic streptococci or *C. perfringens*

Expected Outcome

The patient is free from impaired tissue integrity related to the formation of gas gangrene.
- Does the patient have a high fever?
- Does the patient complain of intense localized pain?
- Is a foul odor present?
- Is tissue crepitant, dark, and cool?

Diagnosis

High risk for impaired tissue integrity related to abscess formation.

Definition

Presence of risk factors for the patient to experience damage to the integumentary or subcutaneous tissue owing to the formation of an abscess.

Risk Factors

- Presence of pus in the wound
- Inadequate wound drainage
- Use of agents such as hydrogen peroxide, 1% povidone-iodine, 0.25% acetic acid, and 0.5% sodium hypochlorite to clean the wound
- Poor wound care

Expected Outcome

The patient is free from impaired tissue integrity related to abscess formation.

- Does the patient show evidence of damage to integumentary or subcutaneous tissue?

Diagnosis

High risk for impaired tissue integrity related to the use of a gelatin sponge.

Definition

Presence of risk factors for the patient to experience nervous, integumentary, and subcutaneous tissue damage related to the use of a gelatin sponge to achieve intraoperative hemostasis.

Risk Factors

- Inappropriate application of a gelatin sponge, resulting in bleeding after closure
- Use during neurosurgery and tendon repairs
- Application to wound edges
- Presence of tissue inflammation

Expected Outcome

The patient is free from damage to nervous, integumentary, or subcutaneous tissue related to the use of a gelatin sponge to achieve intraoperative hemostasis.

- Does the patient show signs of hematoma formation due to vascular oozing?
- Does the patient complain of postoperative pain or neurologic deficit?

Diagnosis

High risk for impaired tissue integrity related to the handling of tissue with instruments during surgery.

Definition

Presence of risk factors for the patient to experience damage to muscle, fascia, subcutaneous tissue, and skin after surgery related to the approximation of tissue and the ligation of blood vessels with suture material.

Risk Factors (Ethicon, 1988, pp. 5, 13)

- Obesity
- Wound infection
- Bleeding disorders
- Nutritional deficiencies
- Poor intraoperative hemostasis
- Inadequate approximation of tissue, resulting in the formation of dead space
- Poor suture knot tying technique; use of an inappropriate suture knot

Expected Outcome

The patient is free from signs of impaired tissue integrity at the wound site.

- Is there swelling at the wound site?
- Is the wound discolored, does it have a serosanguineous discharge?
- Is there excessive pain at the wound site?

Diagnosis

High risk for impaired tissue integrity related to extravasation of IV medication.

Definition

Presence of risk factors for the patient to experience injury to subcutaneous tissue owing to extravasation of the medications and IV solutions.

Risk Factors

- Elderly patients
- Debilitated persons with poor venous access

Expected Outcome

The patient is free from tissue damage related to subcutaneous infiltration of medications and IV fluids.

- Does the IV site have redness, swelling, edema, or other signs of irritation?
- Does the patient complain of pain at the IV site?

Diagnosis

High risk for impaired skin integrity related to improper positioning.

Definition

Presence of risk factors for the patient to experience skin disruption over bony prominences owing to surgical positioning (Gordon, 1987a, p. 84).

Risk Factors

- Prolonged pressure on the bony prominences
- Shearing force
- Pressure on the peripheral nervous or vascular systems
- Physical immobilization, lack of position change for more than $1\frac{1}{2}$ hours
- Inattentive staff leaning on the patient
- Obesity or emaciation
- Change in skin turgor
- Edema
- Pooling of preparation solutions

Expected Outcome

The patient does not show evidence of skin breakdown related to positioning.
  - Are there signs of disruption of skin surfaces or destruction of skin layers, especially over bony prominences? (Gordon, 1987a, p. 88).

Diagnosis

High risk for fluid volume deficit related to the administration of hyperosmotic agents.

Definition

Presence of risk factors for the patient to experience a decrease in circulating volume.

Risk Factors

- Extremes in age and weight
- Presence of other diuretics in the system
- Nausea and vomiting related to the pain of acute angle-closure glaucoma

Expected Outcome

The patient does not experience fluid deficit secondary to the administration of hyperosmotic agents.

- Did the patient experience an unintentional increase in intraocular pressure?
- Was the patient's intraoperative fluid volume maintained?

Diagnosis

High risk for fluid volume deficit related to the use of anticoagulants or antiplatelet agents.

Definition

Presence of risk factors for the patient to experience excessive intraoperative blood loss owing to preoperative or intraoperative use of anticoagulant or antiplatelet agents.

Risk Factors

- Surgical intervention
- Central nervous system trauma
- Pregnancy
- Advanced age and female gender
- Renal insufficiency
- Gastrointestinal disorders
- Alteration in vitamin K absorption
- Tobacco and alcohol use
- Other medications such as aspirin, antihistamines, cough preparations containing guaifensin, and other over-the-counter medications

Expected Outcome

The patient experiences minimal fluid deficit related to anticoagulant therapy.

- Was the patient's hemodynamic status (blood pressure, pulse, and central pressures) maintained within normal limits?

Diagnosis

High risk for fluid volume deficit related to intraoperative or postoperative blood loss.

Definition

Presence of risk factors for the patient to experience intraoperative or postoperative blood loss secondary to alterations in clotting mechanisms.

Risk Factors

- Vitamin K deficiency

- Renal failure
- Myeloproliferative diseases
- Bone marrow replacement
- Severe liver disease, such as cirrhosis and hepatitis
- Malnutrition, obstructive jaundice, antibiotic sterilization of the gastrointestinal tract, or malabsorption
- Mixed coagulation and platelet defects
- Widespread metastatic disease, massive trauma or burns, gram-negative or gram-positive sepsis, and some viral and malarial infections
- Retroplacental hemorrhage
- Incompatible blood products
- Aspirin, dipyridamole, sulfinpyrazone, nonsteroidal anti-inflammatory drugs (sulindac, ibuprofen, piroxicam) and antihistamine use
- Anticoagulant drug use (coumarin [Coumadin] compounds [sodium warfarin] and heparin)
- High doses of dextran
- Snake bites

Expected Outcome

The patient is free from intraoperative or postoperative fluid deficit (bleeding) related to alterations in clotting mechanisms.

- Was there uncontrollable intraoperative bleeding?
- Does the patient have signs of postoperative bleeding, hematoma development, and excessive wound drainage?

Diagnosis

High risk for fluid volume deficit related to intraoperative bleeding.

Definition

Presence of risk factors for the patient to experience significant fluid loss during the intraoperative period owing to hemorrhaging.

Risk Factors

- Type of surgery, the location of the incision, and the duration of the procedure predisposing to bleeding
- Preexisting bleeding disorders and coexisting disease
- Trauma
- Presence of anticoagulant medications in the patient's system (e.g., aspirin, heparin, or warfarin sodium)

Expected Outcome

The patient's fluid volume is maintained during the intraoperative period.

- Is there a decrease in intraoperative urine output?
- Is output greater than intake?
- Is hypotension present?
- Does the patient have an increased pulse rate?
- Is there a decrease in pulse volume/pressure?
- If the patient is awake, is there a change in mental status?
- Is the patient's skin dry to touch?
- Does the patient have dry mucous membranes? (Gordon, 1987a, p. 78)

Diagnosis

High risk for fluid volume excess.

Definition

Presence of risk factors for the patient to experience an increase in body fluid volume from the administration of IV fluids during the perioperative period.

Risk Factors

- Rapid intake of excessive fluid or sodium
- Presence of congestive heart failure, chronic renal failure, or liver disease, resulting in sodium retention
- Stress of surgical intervention
- Cushing syndrome or corticosteroid therapy

Expected Outcome

The patient's fluid volume is maintained.

- Are there signs of edema or effusion?
- Does the patient have a change in mental status?
- Is intake greater than output?
- Is oliguria present?
- Are there changes in specific gravity?
- Does the patient show evidence of shortness of breath, dyspnea, and orthopnea?
- Are the patient's breath sounds normal?
- Does the patient have changes in blood pressure, venous pressure, or pulmonary arterial pressure?
- Is jugular venous distention present?
- Are there decreases in hemoglobin and hematocrit?
- Are electrolytes within normal limits? (Gordon, 1987a, p. 82)

Diagnosis

High risk for fluid volume excess related to the absorption of large amounts of irrigating fluid into the systemic circulation.

Definition

Presence of risk factors for the patient to experience excessive circulation volume owing to absorption of irrigating fluid into the vascular system.

Risk Factors

- History of cardiopulmonary disease
- History of renal dysfunction

Expected Outcome

The patient's hemodynamic status is maintained within normal limits.

- Does the patient have edema?
- Is hypotension or tachycardia present?
- Does the patient complain of angina like pains?
- Does the patient have signs and symptoms of pulmonary congestion?

ELIMINATION PATTERN
Diagnosis

High risk for altered postoperative bowel function.

Definition

Presence of risk factors for the patient to experience prolonged ileus after surgery.

Risk Factors

- Manipulation of intestines intraoperatively
- Decreased activity
- Administration of medications (i.e., narcotics for pain relief)
- Peritonitis
- Septicemia
- Hypovolemia
- Hypokalemia

Expected Outcome

The patient does not experience prolonged adynamic ileus.

- Is the patient's abdomen soft and nondistended?
- Is there an absence of nausea and vomiting?
- Does the patient have a return of bowel sounds in an appropriate amount of time following the surgical procedure?
- Does the patient pass flatus or stool?

ACTIVITY-EXERCISE PATTERN
Diagnosis

High risk for ineffective breathing pattern related to transfer to and from the surgical suite.

Definition

Presence of risk factors that may cause the patient to experience respirations that are insufficient to maintain adequate oxygen supply for cellular requirements during preoperative and postoperative transfer activities (Gordon, 1987a).

Risk Factors (Gordon, 1987a, p. 154)

- Obesity
- Neuromuscular impairment
- Musculoskeletal impairment
- Perceptual or cognitive impairment
- Anxiety
- Preoperative sedation
- Pain
- Improper position of the patient during transfer
- Pregnancy

Expected Outcome

The patient shows no subjective or objective evidence of breathing difficulty.

- Are there verbal or nonverbal expressions of breathing difficulty, orthopnea, dyspnea, shortness of breath, use of accessory muscles, altered chest excursion, tachypnea, cough, and nasal flaring? (Gordon, 1987a, p. 154)

Diagnosis

High risk for ineffective breathing pattern during the postoperative period.

Definition

Presence of risk factors for the patient to experience respirations inadequate to maintain sufficient oxygen supply for cellular requirements during the postoperative period.

Risk Factors

- Ineffective airway clearance
- Stasis of pulmonary secretions
- Aspiration
- Smoking

- Hypoventilation during anesthesia (e.g., deflated lung during pulmonary resection)
- Intraoperative handling of pulmonary tissue, leading to edema or alveolar damage

Expected Outcome

The patient is free from alterations in breathing patterns after surgery.

- Are breath sounds normal?
- Is there resonant percussion over the lung field?
- Is pulse rate within normal limits?
- Is the patient afebrile?
- Is respiratory rate within normal limits (16–20 breaths/minute)?
- Is the patient's cough productive of clear mucus only?
- Is there an absence of pleuritic pain?
- Is the white blood cell count within normal limits?
- Are arterial blood gas values or pulse oximeter readings within normal limits?
- What is the patient's mental status?
- What is the patient's skin color?
- Does the patient have shortness of breath or dyspnea?
- Is there evidence of the use of accessory muscle to breathe, altered chest excursions, tachypnea, nasal flaring, and pursed-lip breathing or a prolonged expiration phase?
- Does the patient make statements indicating respiratory difficulty?
- Does the patient show evidence of labored breathing?
- Are arterial blood gas values within normal limits?
- Are respirations effective? (Gordon, 1987a, p. 154)

Diagnosis

High risk for ineffective breathing pattern related to IV sedation.

Definition

Presence of risk factors for the patient to experience sedative-induced breathing difficulty.

Risk Factors

- Respiratory disorders such as emphysema, asthma, pneumonia, pulmonary tumor, and chronic obstructive pulmonary disease
- Conditions that interfere with normal breathing patterns such as obesity, third trimester of pregnancy, and neuromuscular disorders
- Liver disease that interferes with the metabolism of sedative and narcotics

Expected Outcome

The patient's breathing patterns are maintained during the surgical procedure.
- Does the patient show evidence of wheezing?
- Does the patient show evidence of shallow respirations, dyspnea, hyperventilation, tachypnea, or airway obstruction?
- Are there signs of laryngospasm or bronchospasm?

Diagnosis

High risk for acute pulmonary embolus.

Definition

The presence of risk factors for the patient to experience a deficit in blood supply to the pulmonary circulation related to pulmonary embolus secondary to thrombophlebitis after surgery.

Risk Factors

- Venous stasis from immobility
- Positioning during surgery and in the PACU
- Abdominal distention
- Intraoperative trauma to the pelvic veins

Expected Outcome

The patient is free from deep vein thrombosis.
- Does the patient show evidence of tenderness and pain in the calf?
- Does the patient show evidence of edema in the lower extremities?
- Does the patient have a fever?

Diagnosis

High risk for ineffective airway clearance.

Definition

Presence of risk factors for the patient to experience an inability to clear the airway during the surgical procedure.

Risk Factors (Gordon, 1987a, p. 152)

- Alteration in level of consciousness caused by sedation
- History of sleep apnea or obstruction because of the position of the tongue
- Excessive salivation or the presence of viscous secretions
- Ineffective coughing or an inability to cough due to the nature of the procedure (cataract or other ocular procedure) or lack of

understanding of how and when to breathe deeply and to cough
- Pain or fear of pain that may discourage coughing
- Fatigue, weakness, or drowsiness

Expected Outcome

The patient is free from airway obstruction during the perioperative period.
- Are abnormal breath sounds such as rales, crackles, rhonchi, or wheezes present?
- Does the patient demonstrate a productive cough?
- Is there a change in the patient's rate or depth of respirations?
- Does the patient show evidence of dyspnea at rest or on exertion?
- Does the patient show evidence of tachypnea?
- Is cyanosis present? (Gordon, 1987a, p. 152)

Diagnosis

High risk for ineffective airway clearance during the postoperative period.

Definition

Presence of risk factors for the patient to experience ineffective removal of secretions from the airway because of poor cough after surgery.

Risk Factors

- Bed rest
- Poor cough associated with narcotics, anesthesia, pain, fatigue, tenacious secretions, tracheal edema due to endotracheal intubation, surgical procedures around the trachea such as thyroidectomy and carotid endarterectomy, and abdominal distention
- Presence of a nasogastric tube intraoperatively or postoperatively

Expected Outcome

The patient's airway is maintained.
- Are abnormal breath sounds such as rales, crackles, rhonchi, or wheezes present?
- Does the patient demonstrate a productive cough?
- Is there a change in the patient's rate or depth of respirations?
- Does the patient show evidence of dyspnea at rest or on exertion?
- Does the patient show evidence of tachypnea?
- Is cyanosis present? (Gordon, 1987a, p. 152)

Diagnosis

High risk for altered tissue perfusion related to transfer of the pregnant patient to and from the surgical suite.

Definition

Presence of risk factors that may cause the pregnant patient to experience a decrease in blood supply to vital organs during preoperative and postoperative transfer activities.

Risk Factors

- Interruption of venous flow (e.g., gravid uterus compressing the inferior vena cava
- Supine position of the patient

Expected Outcome

The pregnant patient shows no subjective or objective evidence of altered tissue perfusion.

- Are there verbal or nonverbal statements of discomfort, especially in the lower extremities?
- Is edema present in the lower extremities?

Diagnosis

High risk for decreased cardiac output related to toxicity of local anesthetics.

Definition

Presence of risk factors for the patient to experience a gradual or abrupt fall in blood pressure caused by a toxic response to the local anesthetic.

Risk Factors

- The presence of cardiac depressants can increase the effect of local anesthetics
- Local anesthetics containing epinephrine can precipitate arrhythmias

Expected Outcome

The patient does not experience cardiodepression associated with the administration of local anesthesia.

- Is the patient free from local anesthetic–induced hypotension, tachycardia, and cardiac arrhythmias?

Diagnosis

High risk for decreased cardiac output related to air embolus from IV catheters.

Definition

Presence of risk factors for the patient to experience alterations in cardiac output secondary to an air embolus from the IV catheter.

Risk Factors

- Delivery of fluid under pressure
- Presence of a central IV catheter

Expected Outcome

The patient's cardiac output is maintained.
- Is the patient cyanotic?
- Is the patient hypotensive?
- Is the patient responsive?

Diagnosis

High risk for decreased cardiac output (cardiodepression) related to the administration of local anesthetics.

Definition

Presence of risk factors for the patient to experience cardiodepression during the administration of a local anesthetic.

Risk Factors

- Patient receiving cardiodepressant medications
- Local anesthetics with epinephrine
- Heart block or other cardiac disease

Expected Outcome

The patient's cardiac output is maintained during the surgical procedure.
- Is there gradual or abrupt hypotension?
- Does the patient have good skin color?
- If awake, does the patient complain of feeling faint or dizzy?
- Is tachycardia present?
- Is bradycardia present?

Diagnosis

High risk for alteration in postoperative cardiac rate (tachycardia).

Definition

Presence of risk factors for the patient to experience an increased cardiac rate after surgery.

Risk Factors

- Fever

- Lack of medication routinely taken by the patient, such as digitalis
- Relative hypotension
- Inadequate pain relief
- Apprehension

Expected Outcome

The patient exhibits a cardiac rate within normal limits.
- Is there gradual or abrupt hypotension?
- Does the patient have good skin color?
- Does the patient complain of feeling faint or dizzy?
- Is tachycardia present?
- Is bradycardia present?

Diagnosis

High risk for self-care deficit after surgery.

Definition

Presence of risk factors for the patient to experience a temporary or permanent inability to complete one or more of the following activities of daily living as a result of surgery: feeding, bathing, toileting, dressing, and grooming.

Risk Factors (Gordon, 1987a, p. 132)

- Activity intolerance; decreased strength and endurance related to age, presence of disease, or effect of surgery
- Pain, discomfort
- Uncompensated perceptual-cognitive impairment
- Uncompensated neuromuscular impairment
- Uncompensated musculoskeletal impairment
- Severe anxiety
- Depression
- Treatment modalities such as immobilization (casts and traction) following surgery
- Surgery resulting in loss of limb, sight, hearing, bowel or bladder control
- Lack of functional support systems in the home

Expected Outcome

The patient demonstrates the ability to manage self-care after discharge from the health care facility.
- Does the patient complain of difficulty with eating, bathing, toileting, dressing, and grooming?
- Does the patient require the use of equipment or devices when performing activities of daily living (level I)?

- Does the patient require help from another person, assistance, or supervision when performing activities of daily living (level II)?
- Does the patient require help from another person and equipment or device when performing the activities of daily living (level III)?
- Is the patient dependent and not participating in self-care (level IV)? (Gordon, 1987a, p. 132)

COGNITIVE-PERCEPTUAL PATTERN
Diagnosis

High risk for discomfort or pain related to transfer to and from the surgical suite.

Definition

Presence of risk factors that may cause the patient to experience discomfort or pain during the preoperative or postoperative transfer activities.

Risk Factors
- Existing injury
- Chronic physical disease such as osteoarthritis
- Neuromuscular impairment
- Cognitive or perceptual impairment
- Anxiety
- Surgical wound
- Presence of traction devices
- Equipment malfunction (imbalanced gurney wheels, which cause an uneven ride)
- Careless maneuvering of the gurney or the patient's bed by the transporter

Expected Outcome

The patient shows no subjective or objective evidence of discomfort or pain during the transfer process.
- Are there verbal statements indicating discomfort or pain?
- Does the patient demonstrate nonverbal expressions (e.g., facial masks of pain, guarded movement, crying, or moaning) that indicate discomfort or pain?

Diagnosis

High risk for alteration in comfort related to nausea and vomiting.

Definition

Presence of risk factors for the patient to experience discomfort during the postoperative period due to nausea and vomiting.

Risk Factors

- Visceral irritation
- Postoperative adynamic ileus
- Narcotics
- Anesthetic agents

Expected Outcome (Ulrich et al., 1986)

The patient does not experience postoperative discomfort due to nausea or vomiting.

- Is the patient vomiting?
- Does the patient complain of nausea?

Diagnosis

High risk for alteration in comfort (postoperative pain).

Definition

Presence of risk factors for the patient to experience acute pain after surgery.

Risk Factors

- Surgical incision
- Pressure on nerve endings from edema or purulent substances
- Tissue necrosis from infection
- Chemical irritation from substances used to clean the wound
- Reflex muscle spasm
- Excessive tissue trauma
- Aggressive tissue retraction and manipulation

Expected Outcome

The patient experiences minimal postoperative wound pain.

- Does the patient complain of inadequate pain control?
- Are the patient's facial expressions and body positioning relaxed?
- Does the patient gradually increase activity level?
- Is there a decreased use of pain medications?

Diagnosis

Knowledge deficit related to surgical intervention.

Definition

The patient and/or family members cannot state or explain information regarding the perioperative environment and pertinent aspects of the surgical procedure and the potential physical and psychological effects of surgery and cannot demonstrate coping.

Defining Characteristics (Gordon, 1987a, p. 186)

The patient and/or family members

- Demonstrate less than adequate recall of information about past surgical or invasive procedure experiences or demonstrate misunderstanding, misinterpretation, or misconceptions
- Inaccurately follow through with previous instruction
- Inadequately perform a self-care skill
- Demonstrate inappropriate or exaggerated behaviors such as hysteria, hostility, or apathy

Related Factors (Gordon, 1987a)

- Low readiness for reception of information (anxiety)
- Lack of interest or motivation to learn
- Cognitive limitations
- Uncompensated short-term memory loss
- Inability to use materials or information resources because of such factors as cultural or language differences
- Unfamiliarity with information resources

Expected Outcome

The patient and/or family members demonstrate knowledge concerning the perioperative period.

- Does the patient demonstrate knowledge concerning the perioperative environment and pertinent aspects of the surgical procedure?
- Does the patient demonstrate knowledge concerning the potential physical and psychological effects of surgery?
- Does the patient demonstrate coping mechanisms that can be used in response to surgical intervention?
- Does the patient demonstrate the cognitive, motor, and affective skills necessary to participate in the rehabilitation process after surgery?

SELF-PERCEPTION–SELF-CONCEPT PATTERN
Diagnosis

High risk for fear related to transfer to the surgical suite.

Definition

Presence of risk factors that may cause the patient to experience a feeling of dread related to the impending surgical procedure; the patient who experiences fear related to surgery perceives surgery as a threat or a danger (Gordon, 1987a).

Risk Factors (Gordon, 1987a, p. 198)

- Knowledge excess or deficit
- Perceived inability to control an event
- Anticipation of a negative surgical outcome or prognosis
- Stressful or frightening preoperative preparation routines
- Surgical suite environment
- Stressful interpersonal communication with health care workers
- Stressful interpersonal communication with family members and significant others

Expected Outcome

The patient shows little or moderate subjective or objective evidence of fear.

- Does the patient make verbal statements describing feelings of dread, nervousness, or concerns about the impending surgical procedure?
- Is there an increase in the patient's questioning or information seeking?
- Is the patient restless, with voice tremors or pitch changes, increased verbalization, hand tremors, increased muscle tension, narrowing focus on the impending surgical procedure, diaphoresis, and increased heart and respiratory rate?

Diagnosis

Fear related to the perioperative experience.

Definition

A feeling of dread by the patient because he or she perceives surgery as a threat or danger to the self (Gordon, 1987a, p. 198).

Defining Characteristics (Gordon, 1987a, p. 198)

- The patient describes, with or without assistance, surgery as the focus of threat or danger
- Feelings of dread, nervousness, or concern about the surgical event
- "Verbalized expectation of danger to self
- Increased questioning or information seeking
- Voice tremors, pitch changes
- Increase in quantity of verbalization
- Increased rate of verbalization
- Hand tremor
- Increased muscle tension
- Narrowing focus of attention progressing to fixed focus
- Diaphoresis
- Increased heart rate
- Increased respiratory rate"

Related Factors (Gordon, 1987a, p. 198)

- Knowledge deficit about the impending surgical event or health status
- Perceived inability to control the surgical event or outcome of surgery

Expected Outcome

The patient recognizes and manages fear during the perioperative period.

- Does the patient recognize the presence of fear?
- Is the patient effectively managing the feeling of fear as evidenced by a lack of restlessness, voice tremors or pitch changes, increased verbalization (quantity and rate), hand tremor, increased muscle tension, narrowing focus of attention progressing to a fixed focus, diaphoresis, increased heart rate, increased respiratory rate? (Gordon, 1987a, p. 198)

Diagnosis

High risk for self-esteem disturbance.

Definition

Presence of risk factors for the patient to experience negative feelings or conception of self related to body exposure, particularly during the preparation and draping procedure (Gordon, 1987a, p. 218)

Risk Factors

- Cultural or religious beliefs (i.e., prohibitions against nudity in the presence of the opposite sex)
- Location of operative site such as genitalia or breasts for female patients
- Type of anesthesia (local, regional, or spinal)
- Derogatory comments or joking by the staff concerning the patient's appearance, weight, or physical condition
- Mixed gender of the staff
- Unnecessary traffic flow in the operating room

Expected Outcome

The patient is free from negative feelings or conception of self during the preparation and draping for the surgical procedure.

- Did the patient make verbal expressions of anxiety or shame during the operative preparation or draping procedure?
- Did the patient demonstrate restlessness, increased perspiration, facial tension, clenched hands, or shakiness in the extremities? (Gordon, 1987a, p. 202)

Diagnosis

Anticipatory anxiety (mild, moderate, or severe) related to the perioperative experience.

Definition

Patients experiencing anticipatory anxiety have an "increased level of arousal associated with a perceived future threat (unfocused) to the self or significant relationships" (Gordon, 1987a, p. 200).

Defining Characteristics (Gordon, 1987a, pp. 200, 202)

- Surgical intervention perceived by the patient "as a threat to physical or psychosocial self (unfocused)"
- Verbalization of apprehension, uncertainty, fear, distress, or worry
- Verbalization of painful and persistent feelings of increased helpless, inadequacy, regret
- Expressions of concern (change in life events)
- Fear of unspecified consequences
- Overexcited, rattled, jittery, scared state
- Restlessness, focus on self, insomnia, increased perspiration
- Increased wariness, glancing about, poor eye contact, facial tension, voice quivering
- Increased tension, foot shuffling, hand/arm movements, trembling, hand tremor, shakiness

Related Factors (Gordon, 1987a, p. 202)

- Surgical intervention perceived by the patient "as a threat to self concept, health status, socioeconomic status, role functioning, interaction patterns, or environment"
- Perceived threat of death related to the surgical experience
- Unconscious conflict (essential values, life goals) triggered by surgical intervention

Expected Outcome

The patient identifies and manages anticipatory anxiety.
- Does the patient recognize the presence of anticipatory anxiety?
- Is the patient effectively managing anticipatory anxiety?

Diagnosis

High risk for body image disturbance related to anticipated changes in body appearance or function secondary to surgical intervention.

Definition

Presence of risk factors for the patient to experience negative feelings or perceptions about characteristics, functions, or limits of the body or a body part as a result of surgical intervention (Gordon, 1987a, p. 220).

Risk Factors
- Surgery for removal of body part significant to sexual identity
- Surgery resulting in a change in the appearance of body parts visible to others (face, neck, hands)
- Amputation
- Verbalization by the patient that he or she will experience difficulty in integrating the impending body change.
- Verbalization by the patient that the body will be imperfect following surgery.

Expected Outcome
The patient acknowledges the presence of body image disturbance after surgery and engages in functional coping behaviors.
- Has the patient acknowledged the presence of body image disturbance?
- Is the patient demonstrating evidence of functional coping behaviors?

ROLE-RELATIONSHIP PATTERN
Diagnosis
Anticipatory grieving related to the effect of surgery.

Definition
Expectation by the patient that he or she will experience a disruption in familiar patterns or significant relationships concerning other people, possessions, job, status, home, ideals, and parts and processes of the body after surgery (Gordon, 1987a, p. 228).

Defining Characteristics (Gordon, 1987a, p. 228)
- Surgery for removal of body part significant to sexual identity
- Surgery resulting in a change in the appearance of body parts visible to others (face, neck, hands)
- Amputation
- "Verbal expression of distress at potential (anticipated) loss
- Anger
- Sadness, sorrow, crying
- Crying at frequent intervals, choked feeling
- Change in eating habits
- Alteration in sleep or dream patterns
- Alteration in activity level
- Altered libido
- Idealization of anticipated loss

- Developmental regression
- Alterations in concentration or pursuit of tasks"

Related Factors (Gordon, 1987a, p. 228)

- Expected loss or change related to anticipated surgical result

Expected Outcome

The patient recognizes the presence of anticipatory grief and engages in a functional grieving process.

- Does the patient acknowledge the presence of anticipatory grief?
- Is the patient engaged in a functional grieving process?

COPING–STRESS TOLERANCE PATTERN
Diagnosis

Ineffective individual coping related to the stress of impending surgery.

Definition

Impairment of a patient's abilities to use adaptive behaviors and problem-solving techniques for meeting life's demands and roles during the perioperative period. The patient's usual patterns of coping with stressful life situations are insufficient to control.

Defining Characteristics (Gordon 1987a, p. 284)

- Verbalization of inability to cope
- Inability to ask for help
- Inability to effectively solve problems
- Anxiety, fear, anger, irritability, tension
- Presence of life stress such as a major surgical experience or disease process
- Inability to meet role expectations such as a permanent or temporary loss of employment as a consequence of surgery
- Inability to meet basic needs
- Alteration in societal participation
- Destructive behavior toward self and others
- Inappropriate or ineffective use of defense mechanisms
- Change in usual communication patterns
- Excess food intake, alcohol consumption, smoking
- Digestive, bowel, appetite disturbance; chronic fatigue or sleep pattern disturbance

Related Factors (Gordon 1987a, p. 284)

- Situational crises such as surgery
- Personal vulnerability

- Knowledge deficit concerning surgery
- Problem-solving skills deficit

Expected Outcome

The patient demonstrates the ability to cope with the stresses associated with surgical intervention.

- Does the patient verbalize an inability to cope?
- Does the patient refuse to ask for help?
- Is the patient's problem solving ability impaired?
- Does the patient show evidence of anxiety, fear, anger, irritability, or tension?
- Is the patient unable to meet role expectations?
- Is the patient meeting basic needs?
- Does the patient show evidence of destructive behavior toward self or others?
- Is the patient using inappropriate defense mechanisms?
- Are there changes in the patient's usual communication patterns?
- Does the patient attempt to manipulate verbally?
- Is there evidence of an excess in food intake, alcohol consumption, or smoking?
- Does the patient complain of digestive, bowel, or appetite disturbances?
- Does the patient complain of chronic fatigue or sleep pattern disturbance? (Gordon, 1987a, p. 284)

Diagnosis

Ineffective family coping: disabling related to surgery and the surgical outcome for a loved one.

Definition

Behavior demonstrated by a significant other that disables the significant other's or the patient's ability to perform the tasks essential to either person's adaptation to the process or outcome of the surgical experience (Gordon, 1987a, p. 300).

Defining Characteristics (Gordon 1987a, p. 300)

- Neglectful care of the patient in regard to basic human needs or treatment of illness
- Distortion of reality regarding the patient's health problem, including extreme denial about existence or severity
- Intolerance
- Rejection
- Abandonment
- Desertion

- Carrying on usual routines and disregarding patient's needs
- Taking on illness signs of client
- Decisions and actions by family that are detrimental to economic or social well-being
- Agitation, depression, aggression, hostility
- Impaired restructuring of a meaningful life for self, impaired individuation, prolonged overconcern for patient
- Neglectful relationship with other family members
- Patient's development of helpless, inactive dependence

Related Factors (Gordon 1987a, p. 302)

- Chronically unexpressed guilt/anxiety/hostility/etc. (significant other)
- Dissonant discrepancy of coping styles (for dealing with adaptive task by the significant person and patient or among significant persons)
- Highly ambivalent family relationships
- Arbitrary handling of family's resistance to treatment (which tends to solidify defensiveness as it fails to deal adequately with underlying anxiety)

Expected Outcome

Ineffective family coping does not disable the patient's or significant other's ability to address the tasks essential to the process or outcome of the surgical experience.

- Does the patient or significant other comply with preoperative and postoperative instructions?
- Does the patient or significant other comply with the treatment regimen after surgery?
- Are there signs that the family shows intolerance, rejection, abandonment, or desertion of the patient?
- Is patient psychosomaticism present?
- Are there signs of agitation, depression, aggression, or hostility from the family to the patient?
- Does a family member take on the signs and symptoms of the patient's illness?
- Are there signs of neglectful relationship with other family members?
- Does the patient become helpless and inactively dependent?
- Is there evidence of a distortion of reality regarding the patient's illness, including denial of the existence or severity of the illness? (Gordon, 1987a, p. 300)

CRITICAL COMPETENCIES FOR THE PERIOPERATIVE NURSE

This section provides a step-by-step discussion of how to
- Transfer a patient during the perioperative period
- Provide patient and family education
- Create and maintain a sterile field
- Perform sponge, sharps, and instrument counts
- Provide instruments, equipment, and supplies
- Administer drugs and solutions
- Physiologically monitor the patient
- Monitor and control the environment
- Position the patient
- Handle cultures and specimens

The Association of Operating Room Nurses (AORN) *Competency Statements in Perioperative Nursing* were used as a framework for this section (AORN, 1992, *II*:2–4—2–12). Two competencies—positioning the patient and handling cultures and specimens—were added to the list identified by AORN.

TRANSFERRING THE PATIENT

The perioperative nurse demonstrates competency to transfer the patient by
- Correctly identifying the patient
- Performing or directing the transfer of the patient from the nursing unit to the surgical suite holding area
- Admitting the patient to the surgical suite
- Performing or directing the transfer of the patient from the surgical suite holding area to the operating room (OR)
- Assisting with the transfer of the patient from the OR to the postanesthesia care unit (PACU)

- Performing or directing the transfer of the patient from the OR to the nursing unit after local anesthesia
- Performing or directing the transfer of the patient with special needs
- Performing or directing necessary documentation and verbal communication

Considerations

- Use only qualified personnel, such as the perioperative nurse, the surgical technologist, and the orderly or nursing assistant, who are trained to implement appropriate safety measures to perform transfer activities.
- Ensure that all transfer equipment is functioning according to manufacturer's specifications.
- Ensure that transfer personnel have knowledge of proper body mechanics.

Transferring the Patient to the Surgical Suite Holding Area

Supplies and Equipment

- Gurney (wheeled stretcher) with functional side rails
- Safety strap
- IV pole
- Emesis basin
- Oxygen tank
- Cover sheet
- Head cover for the patient
- Patient pickup slip

Preparing for the Transfer

- After receiving the patient transfer assignment, review the perioperative nursing care plan to check nursing orders concerning transportation, equipment requirements, and planned patient care activities during the transfer.
- Obtain the transfer slip (pickup slip), which identifies the patient by name, hospital number, and location. Don a cover gown and remove headgear and shoe covers. Note the time of departure from the surgical suite.
- Obtain the needed transportation equipment and check for proper functioning.
- Proceed to the designated nursing unit.

Arriving on the Nursing Unit

- After arriving on the nursing unit, report to the charge nurse and ask if the patient is ready to go to surgery.
- Request assistance from unit personnel.

Reviewing the Patient's Chart

- Before entering the patient's room, review the patient's chart.
  1. Check the consent form to ensure that it is signed and witnessed according to hospital policy and procedure.
  2. Check the preoperative check list to ensure that jewelry has been removed, the patient has voided and has had nothing by mouth, and all prostheses (dentures, hearing aid, etc.) have been removed.
  3. Check the chart for x-ray films, electrocardiogram, and laboratory reports.
  4. Check for other routine preoperative reports specific to the institution.

Arriving at the Patient's Room

- Unit nursing personnel should accompany the transporter to the patient's room to identify the location of the patient on the unit, perform the preliminary identification of the patient, and assist with the transfer process.
- After arriving in the patient's room, allow the unit nurse to tell the patient that the transporter is to take him or her to the surgical suite.

Alert and Oriented Patient

- Upon entering the patient's room or holding cubicle, greet the patient by her or his full name. Introduce yourself to the patient and ask the patient to state her or his name and the surgical procedure she or he is having done.
- As the patient states her or his name, read the name on the transfer slip obtained from the surgical suite. Do a second identity check by comparing the name and hospital number on the transfer slip with the name and number on the patient's identification bracelet. Do a third check by checking the transfer slip and the patient's chart.
- Check the consent form again to ensure that the procedure identified on the consent form is the same as that identified by the patient.
- If discrepancies are noted, call the surgical suite for guidance.

Child

- The steps described above for identifying an alert and oriented adult patient must be followed when identifying a child.
- Establish initial contact simultaneously with the child and the parents or legal guardian.
- The parents or legal guardian signed the consent authorizing the surgical procedure; therefore, ask the parents or legal guardian the child's name and the procedure being done.

- If the child's development permits, also ask the child questions.
- If the parent or legal guardian is unavailable, rely on the unit nursing staff to identify the patient. This does not negate the need to check the transfer slip against the patient's hospital bracelet and chart.

Comatose and Disoriented Patient

- With modifications, follow the steps for identifying an alert adult when identifying the comatose and disoriented patient. If present, family members or a significant other should be asked to identify the patient.
- In the absence of family members or a significant other, rely on the unit nursing staff or other personnel, such as a surgeon or a police officer if the patient is in the emergency room, to identify the patient. Again, it is important to compare the transfer slip with the patient's hospital bracelet and chart.

Transferring the Patient to the Gurney

- After explaining what is going to happen, cover the patient with a sheet or blanket.
- Position the gurney adjacent to the bed and lock the wheels of the bed and the gurney.
- Stand next to the gurney and have the unit nursing personnel stand opposite, next to the bed.
- Raise the bed to the level of the gurney.
- Tell the patient to move from the bed to the gurney, buttocks first, shoulders second, and feet last. During the transfer, have the unit nursing personnel stabilize the bed by leaning against it. At the same time, lean against the gurney.
- After the patient is on the gurney, raise the side rails and fasten the safety belt across the patient's thighs.
- Tell the patient to keep fingers, hands, arms, and legs, including the knees, away from the side rails.

Transporting the Patient to the Surgical Suite

- If family members or significant others are present, ask them to accompany the patient to the surgical suite entrance.
- Push the gurney, with the patient's feet first, through corridors.
- When turning corners, ensure that obstacles or people are not unexpectedly encountered.
- If an elevator is used, pull the gurney in headfirst.
- After arriving at the designated floor, pull the gurney out of the elevator. While pulling the gurney out, hold the elevator doors back to prevent their inadvertent closure on the gurney.

- On arrival in the surgical suite, if visitors are not permitted in the holding area, allow them to interact with the patient before he or she enters the suite.
- Tell or show significant others where to wait while the patient is having surgery. Tell them that the surgeon will be informed that they are in the waiting room so that he or she may speak to them after the surgical procedure.
- Before entering the surgical suite, remove your cover gown and don shoe covers and headgear.
- If the surgical suite doors are not automatic, open one of the doors, lean against it, and pull the gurney footfirst through the doorway.
- If the doors are automatic, allow them to open completely before the gurney is moved through the doorway.
- When in the holding area, lock the wheels of the gurney and tell the holding area nurse and the patient care coordinator of the surgical suite that the patient has arrived.
- Before leaving the patient, document on the patient's chart the method of transfer, who transported the patient, safety measures used, and the time that the patient arrived in the surgical suite.

Admitting the Patient to the Surgical Suite Holding Area
Supplies
- Perioperative documents
- Laboratory request slips
- Patient's hospital card
- Blood pressure cuff and sphygmomanometer
- Temperature probes and recording devices
- Oxygen and associated delivery devices
- Suction devices
- Emesis basins
- Urinals and bedpans
- Warm blankets
- Preparation equipment such as depilatory, shaving cream, and razors
- IV needles, tubing, and bags
- Electrocardiographic monitors and pulse oximeters

Reviewing the Patient's Chart
- Greet the patient and put him or her at ease.
- Review the chart for completeness and the patient data card for accuracy.
- Determine whether the patient has voided, removed jewelry and prostheses, and received prescribed preoperative medications.

- Check the chart for prescribed test reports and the history and physical examination findings.
- Ask the patient about allergies.
- Validate nothing by mouth status by asking the patient the last time he or she had something to eat or drink.
- Investigate items on the checklist that are not initialed as completed before the transfer to the surgical suite and take corrective action.
- Determine whether the consent form has been completed according to hospital policy.
- If hospital protocols have not been followed, barring emergency situations, postpone surgery until consent can be obtained.
- Review the preoperative orders to determine whether blood or blood products have been ordered for the patient.
- If blood has been ordered, check with the patient care coordinator to ensure that the blood is present in the surgical suite blood refrigerator. If the blood is not present, call the laboratory to ensure that the order has been received and to check blood availability.

Preparing the Intraoperative Paperwork

- Prepare paperwork for intraoperative documentation before the patient is transferred to the OR.
- Depending on the surgical procedure and hospital policy and procedure, use the data card to stamp the anesthetic record, operative report, intraoperative nursing record (if separate from operative report), charge slips, labels, and slips from pathology, laboratory, and radiology departments.

Transferring the Patient From the Holding Area to the Operating Room

Supplies and Equipment

- OR bed
- Draw (lift) sheet
- Arm boards
- Safety straps for the legs and arms
- IV poles
- Warm sheets
- Headrest

Preparing for the Transfer

- After ensuring that all surgical team members are ready to receive the patient, proceed to the holding area and check with the nurse about the status of the patient.
- Greet the patient and tell her or him that she or he is to be transported to the OR.

- After verifying the patient's identity, allergies, and nothing by mouth status and the planned procedure, check the chart for the consent form and the presence of laboratory and radiology department reports.

Transporting the Patient to the Operating Room

- Unlock the wheels of the gurney and transport the patient to the OR feet first.
- On entering the OR, announce to the surgical team that the patient is entering the room.
- Introduce the patient to the staff in the room.
- After lowering the side rail next to the OR bed, position the gurney adjacent to the bed and lock the wheels of the gurney. The wheels of the OR bed should have already been locked; however, they should be checked before the patient is moved.
- Lower the other side rail.

Mobile Patient

- Stand next to the gurney and ask the anesthetist or the orderly to stand on the opposite side of the OR bed to protect the patient from falling off the bed during transfer.
- If a blanket was placed around the patient during transfer to the surgical suite, remove it, leaving only the cover sheet over the patient.
- Secure the IV bag to the IV pole located at the head of the bed.
- If the patient has drainage devices, detach from the gurney and place them on the patient or hold them.
- Ask the patient to move to the OR bed, moving buttocks first, shoulders second, and feet last.
- Maintain the patient's modesty by keeping the cover sheet in place during the transfer.

Immobile Patient

- Depending on the patient's size, at least four people are needed to move the immobile patient.
- The lifters (the circulating nurse and assistants) place themselves on each side of the OR bed and one at the foot of the bed.
- The anesthetist remains at the head of the bed.
- Place the patient's arms across the chest. Have the side lifters position themselves as close to the OR bed and gurney as possible. Their legs should be apart, one ahead of the other.
- Have the side lifters roll the drawsheet up against the patient's side and grasp the sheet up against the patient.
- The anesthetist directs the transfer and controls the patient's head. Do not move the patient until the patient's airway is stabilized.

- The anesthetist counts aloud to ensure that all lifters begin the transfer in a synchronized motion.
- The foot lifter crosses the patient's legs at the ankles and grasps the ankles with both hands. The lifter stands erect at the foot of the gurney and prepares to lift the legs. On the count of the anesthetist, the lifter moves one step in the direction the patient is being moved. The patient's ankles are lifted and gently lowered onto the OR bed.
- The side lifter next to the gurney places her or his dominant leg approximately 6 to 8 inches behind the nondominant leg. Both legs should be slightly bent. Because the dominant leg is usually stronger, the lifter's own body weight should be shifted to the dominant leg. This makes it easier for the lifter to bear the patient's weight during the transfer.
- The lifter maintains her or his upper torso in a straight upright position. When the transfer begins, the lifter lifts the patient by straightening the legs, lifting the drawsheet under the patient, and slightly walking forward or shifting the weight from her or his back leg (the dominant leg) to the front leg.
- During the maneuver, the lifter bends slightly at the waist as the patient moves away from her or him, simultaneously keeping the upper torso straight. The patient is gently lowered onto the OR bed.
- The side lifter next to the OR bed places her or his dominant leg approximately 6 to 8 inches in front of the nondominant leg. Both legs should be slightly bent. As the transfer begins, the side lifter lifts the patient by straightening her or his legs, lifting the drawsheet, and taking one step backward or shifting the weight from her or his front leg (the dominant leg) to the back leg. Simultaneously, while shifting the weight, she or he straightens at the waist and keeps the upper torso in an upright position. The patient is gently lowered onto the OR bed.

Securing the Patient on the Operating Room Bed

- After the patient is on the OR bed, center the patient's hips and check the body alignment of the patient's shoulders, abdomen, and feet along the length of the bed.
- Place a safety strap across the patient's thighs, approximately 2 inches above the knees, and secure.
- Check to ensure that the strap is not too tight or too loose by placing one hand between the thighs and the strap. The strap should not be so tight as to prevent the hand's being placed between it and the thighs.
- Place the patient's hands and arms on the arm boards and secure with arm straps.

Transferring the Patient From the Operating Room to the Postanesthesia Care Unit

Supplies and Equipment

- Recovery bed with an IV pole and functional side rails
- Oxygen tank with delivery valve and tubing and at least 500 to 1000 pounds/square inch (psi) in the tank
- Oral airway
- Warm sheet and blanket
- Patient body roller

Preparing to Transfer the Patient From the Operating Room Bed

- Four people are needed as described for transferring the immobile patient to the recovery bed.
- Place the patient's arms across the chest.
- The side lifter on the side opposite the recovery bed holds the patient's arms across the chest.
- Remove the arm boards from the bed and move away from the bed, thus enabling the recovery bed to be placed adjacent to the OR bed.
- Lock the wheels of the recovery bed.
- If the patient is unresponsive or unable to control his or her arms, the lifter on the opposite side of the OR bed from the recovery bed ensures that the patient's arms remain across the chest.
- Ensuring that the IV solutions are not lowered below the level of the patient's heart, move the IV bags to the IV pole on the recovery bed.
- Move drainage tubes to the recovery bed.
- Exercise care to ensure that IV bags are not elevated above the tube exit sites.
- Remove the safety strap.

Transferring the Patient to the Recovery Bed

Mobile Patient

- If the patient is alert, the anesthetist directs the patient to move to the bed, buttocks first, shoulders second, and feet last.
- Lean against the recovery bed and assists the patient as he or she moves and ensure that modesty is maintained.
- After the patient moves to the recovery bed, center and align the patient and raise the side rails.
- If indicated, the anesthetist opens the valve on the oxygen tank and secures the mask or nasal cannula.

Immobile Patient OR Bed Tilt Technique

- For this transfer technique, personnel stand next to the OR bed and recovery bed as described for transferring the immobile patient to the OR bed.
- Raise the OR bed above the level of the recovery bed.
- The side lifter standing next to the OR bed reaches across the patient and grasps the drawsheet. The sheet is wrapped over the patient and the lifter holds the patient in position while the OR bed is tilted.
- The recovery bed is moved slightly away from the OR bed to allow the anesthetist to operate the lever and thus tilt the bed. The bed is tilted toward the recovery bed.
- After the OR bed is tilted as much as possible, the recovery bed is moved back against the OR bed. The circulating nurse stands next to the recovery bed.
- The side lifter holding the patient releases the end of the drawsheet that was used to hold the patient in place. The circulating nurse reaches across the recovery bed to grasp the free end of the drawsheet and places one foot in front of the other. During this maneuver, the circulating nurse bends slightly at the waist and keeps the upper torso straight.
- On the anesthetist's count, the circulating nurse pulls the drawsheet and the patient toward the recovery bed. While doing this, the circulating nurse shifts her or his body weight from the front foot to the back foot and simultaneously raises the upper torso, which is kept straight.
- The side lifter on the opposite side places one foot in front of the other and shifts his or her weight to the back foot. He or she pulls the draw sheet taut under the patient and positions his or her hands against the patient, one at the shoulders and the other at the hips. On the anesthetist's count, the lifter shifts his or her weight to the front foot, bends slightly at the waist while keeping the upper torso straight, and moves the patient down the incline created by the tilted OR bed to the recovery bed. During this maneuver, the anesthetist moves the patient's head and the lifter at the foot of the bed moves the patient's legs and feet.

Roller Technique

- Transfer personnel stand next to the recovery bed and the OR bed as described for transferring the immobile patient to the OR bed. The safety strap is removed by the circulating nurse.
- The side lifter next to the OR bed reaches across the patient and grasps the drawsheet. With permission from the anesthetist, the sheet is pulled up and the patient rolls toward the lifter.

- After the patient is placed on his or her side, the circulating nurse, who is standing next to the recovery bed, places the body roller under the drawsheet as far as possible. The roller should not extend above the head or foot of the recovery bed. It should be placed between the patient's shoulders and thighs.
- The patient is then lowered onto the roller.
- The circulating nurse stands with one leg slightly ahead of the other and reaches across the recovery bed and grasps the drawsheet.
- Care should be exercised to ensure that the circulator's upper torso remains straight and does not bend along the spine during the transfer process.
- On the anesthetist's count, the circulator steps backward and slightly raises her or his upper torso while pulling the drawsheet toward her or him.
- The lifter on the other side of the OR bed also moves the patient on the anesthetist's count. This lifter takes one step forward while bending slightly at the waist. Like the circulating nurse, the lifter keeps his or her torso straight.
- The lifter then moves the patient at the shoulder and hip over the roller to the recovery bed.
- The anesthetist moves the patient's head while the lifter at the foot of the OR bed moves the patient's feet.
- After the transfer is complete, the lifter next to the OR bed positions himself or herself next to the recovery bed, opposite the circulating nurse.
- On the anesthetist's count, the roller is removed by the lifter as the circulating nurse rolls the patient toward her or him with the drawsheet. After the roller is removed, the drawsheet is pushed under the patient as far as possible.
- The circulating nurse then rolls the patient back on her or his back and the drawsheet is removed.
- At this time, residue preparation solution, blood, and other secretions are removed with a warm wet towel or sponge. The patient is then dried and covered with a warm blanket. Side rails are raised, and the patient is transferred to the PACU.

Transferring the Patient to the Postanesthesia Care Unit

- After collecting the chart, nursing notes, and x-ray films, accompany the patient to the PACU.
- Transport the patient feetfirst.
- During the transfer, pull the recovery bed and help the anesthetist to maneuver the bed.
- In the PACU, give a report to the postanesthesia nurse. At a minimum, the report should include the patient's condition, the

intraoperative nursing care provided, and the location of dressing and drainage devices.

Transferring the Patient From the Surgical Suite to the Nursing Unit After Local Anesthesia

Supplies and Equipment

- Gurney with functional side rails
- Safety strap
- IV pole
- Emesis basin
- Warm covering for the patient

Preparing for the Transfer

- After transferring and securing the patient to the gurney, collect the chart, nursing notes, and x-ray films and unlock the gurney wheels.
- If transport to the nursing unit is delayed, transport the patient to an appropriate holding area to await transfer back to the nursing unit.

Giving a Patient Status Report to the Nursing Unit Nurse

- Contact the unit nurse by telephone. Information given to the unit nurse includes the patient's condition, an overview of vital signs during the procedure, the medications given during surgery, and the dosage, drainage devices, and physician's orders that must be implemented immediately after the patient returns to the nursing unit.

Transferring the Patient to the Nursing Unit

- Before departure, assess the patient to determine whether a registered nurse should accompany the patient to the unit.
- The patient is transferred as described for transporting the patient to the surgical suite holding area.
- After arrival on the nursing unit, ensure that nursing personnel know that the patient has returned to the unit.

Transferring the Patient with Special Needs

Supplies and Equipment

- Gurney with functional side rails
- Safety strap
- IV pole
- Cover sheet and a head cover for the patient
- Warm infant transport vehicle for neonates
- Crib for young children
- Oxygen tanks with delivery devices
- Portable monitor and defibrillator unit

Intensive Care Patient

- A perioperative nurse or an intensive care nurse should accompany all patients from the intensive care unit to the surgical suite. If the patient requires respiratory assistance, an anesthetist or a respiratory therapist should also accompany the patient.
- Before transporting the patient from the intensive care unit, contact the intensive care unit nurse to determine transfer needs.
- After collecting the appropriate equipment and ensuring its proper functioning, proceed to the intensive care unit with an orderly and an anesthetist or a respiratory therapist, if warranted.
- Before departing from the intensive care unit, coordinate with the surgical suite patient care coordinator to ensure that patient will immediately be taken into the designated OR on arrival.
- Do not begin the transfer until the OR is ready.

Patient With Major Orthopedic Injuries

- Before transporting the patient with an orthopedic injury, make an assessment to determine the extent of injury, the traction or immobilization devices in use, and the appropriate vehicle for transfer.
- Generally, patients with extensive injuries and multiple skeletal support devices are transported to the surgical suite in their orthopedic bed.
- Since orthopedic beds with traction devices are not designed for transporting patients to the surgical suite, and therefore are not easy to handle, use additional personnel to move the bed through hospital corridors and onto elevators.
- When transferring the patient with traction devices, ensure that the transfer is accomplished without compromise of the patient's traction induced skeletal alignment.

Neonate

- Like the intensive care patient, the neonate is taken directly to the OR.
- Make a preoperative assessment to determine the extent of care required.
- Use a warmed infant transport vehicle during the transfer.
- Depending on the condition of the patient, the perioperative nurse, the pediatrician, or the anesthetist accompanies the patient to the surgical suite.
- Equipment needed for the neonate may include an oxygen tank with the appropriate delivery equipment, a portable monitor and defibrillator, and an IV infusion device. The perioperative nurse should ensure that the neonate's parents know that they may accompany the patient to the surgical suite if they desire.

- The neonate is not transferred until the OR is warmed and prepared for surgery.

Toddlers

- Transport toddlers and other children who are difficult to restrain in a crib with a bubble top and side rails up.
- Have the parent accompany the child to the surgical suite.
- If possible, the parent may carry the child while the transporter pushes the crib.
- On arrival in the surgical suite holding area, parents may stay with the patient until the circulating nurse is ready to take him or her into the OR.

PATIENT AND FAMILY TEACHING

The perioperative nurse demonstrates competency to provide patient and family teaching by

- Identifying the patient's and the family's learning needs
- Assessing the patient's and the family's readiness to learn
- Providing instruction on the basis of identified needs
- Determining the effectiveness of teaching
- Communicating and documenting teaching (AORN, 1992).

Identifying the Learning Needs

- Ask open-ended questions.
- Look for verbal and nonverbal cues.
- Ask the patient and the family what they know about the impending surgical intervention. Do not assume that a lack of questions by the patient or family indicates knowledge of the impending surgical event.
- Identify knowledge concerning surgical routines, nothing-by-mouth status requirements, deep breathing, expansion breathing, splinting of the wound site, coughing, postoperative leg exercises, and discharge instructions.

Assessing the Readiness to Learn

- Determine the patient's and the family's knowledge, attitudes, and self-care skills relative to surgical intervention.
- Ask about past experiences related to the health problem.
- Identify obstacles to health learning.
- Determine level of anxiety (low levels of anxiety enhance learning, whereas moderate and high levels inhibit learning).
- Ask about the patient's and family's educational background (a person's use of vocabulary and ability to communicate can provide clues to the educational background).

- Determine the extent of patient orientation and short term memory capability.
- Assess the patient's physical condition (levels of discomfort, energy, alertness, and so on).
- Determine the patient's developmental level (intellectual and emotional).
- Check for the presence of mental, physical, or educational handicaps (language barrier, sensory deficits).
- Determine the extent of the patient's motivation and attitude (consider the patient's perception of disease or condition and its seriousness) (Toth, 1983).

Providing Instruction Based on Identified Needs

- Provide an overview of expected procedures and events, such as a description of the environment, the sequence of events, and procedures that the patient will experience.
- Describe behaviors that the patient is expected to demonstrate, such as a preoperative shower and nothing-by-mouth status.
- Describe probable alterations in comfort level, such as wound pain, soreness from retractors, and sore throat after general anesthesia with endotracheal intubation.
- Provide strategies for reducing pain and discomfort, such as requesting pain medication and ice chips.
- Describe probable tactile, auditory, and visual sensations that the patient will experience while in the operating room.
- Explain potentially frightening equipment that the patient will see or hear while in the operating room.
- Describe postoperative behaviors that the patient is expected to demonstrate, such as passive exercises, ambulation, deep breathing and coughing, dressing care, and resumption of diet.
- Teach the patient to perform such skills as deep breathing, expansion breathing, wound splinting and coughing, passive leg exercises, and ambulation.

Determining the Effectiveness of Teaching

Teaching has been effective if the patient and/or family members can demonstrate knowledge of the perioperative environment and pertinent aspects of the operative procedure. The patient and/or family members should be able to

- State the time when surgery is scheduled
- State the unit to which the patient will return after surgery
- List monitoring and therapeutic devices or materials most likely to be used during the postoperative period
- State the location of the family waiting areas
- Ask questions about the impending surgery

- Perform expected behaviors such as taking a preoperative shower and maintaining nothing by mouth status (Kneedler and Dodge, 1987)

Teaching has been effective if the patient and family members can demonstrate knowledge of the potential physical and psychological effects of surgery. The patient and/or family members should be able to

- Describe in their own words the anticipated physical and psychological effects of surgical intervention
- Express their feelings regarding surgical intervention and its expected outcomes (Kneedler and Dodge, 1987)

Teaching has been effective if the patient and family members can demonstrate knowledge of coping mechanisms that can be used in response to surgical intervention. The patient and/or family members should be able to

- Verbalize expectations about pain relief
- State the measures that can be taken to alleviate pain
- Identify family and community support systems (Kneedler and Dodge, 1987)

Teaching has been effective if the patient and family members can demonstrate knowledge about how to participate in the rehabilitation process after surgery. The patient and/or family members should be able to

- Cite the reasons for each of the preoperative instructions provided and exercises explained or practiced
- Demonstrate turning, coughing, deep breathing, incision splinting, passive leg exercising, and ambulating
- Describe anticipated steps in postoperative activity resumption (Kneedler and Dodge, 1987)

Documentation and Communication Procedures

- Communicate patient and family teaching to appropriate health care team members.
- Document patient and family teaching in the patient's record.

CREATING AND MAINTAINING A STERILE FIELD

The perioperative nurse demonstrates competency to create and maintain a sterile field by

- Donning surgical attire
- Performing the surgical hand scrub
- Donning sterile gown and gloves
- Preparing a sterile field
- Performing preoperative skin preparation
- Draping the patient and equipment

Critical Considerations for Creating and Maintaining a Sterile Field
Principles of Aseptic Technique

- Only sterile items are used within the sterile field.
- A sterile barrier must be considered contaminated after it has been penetrated.
- The edges of a sterile package or container are considered contaminated after it is opened.
- Gowns are considered sterile only in front from shoulder level to table level and the sleeves to 2 inches above the elbow.
- Only the horizontal surface of a table is considered sterile.
- Sterile persons and items touch only sterile areas. Nonsterile persons or items touch only nonsterile areas.
- Movement within or around the sterile field must not contaminate that field.
- All items and areas of doubtful sterility must be considered contaminated (AORN, 1992, *III*:2–1—2–5).

Donning Surgical Attire (AORN, 1992, *III*:3–1—3–5)
General Considerations

- Before entering the semirestricted and restricted areas of the OR, don proper surgical attire. The surgical suite is divided into three designated areas:
  1. The unrestricted area includes a control point where both OR personnel and other members of the health care facility communicate. Street clothes are permitted in this area.
  2. The semirestricted area includes the peripheral support areas (i.e., hallways, storage areas, processing areas, OR offices). Scrub attire and caps are required in semirestricted areas.
  3. The restricted area includes the area where surgical procedures are performed and where unwrapped supplies are sterilized (i.e., clean core, substerile areas). Scrub attire, caps, and masks are required in this area (AORN, 1992, *III*:3–1 and 22–1—22–3).

Supplies and Equipment

- Scrub top and pants
- Long-sleeved warm-up jacket for unscrubbed personnel
- Disposable bouffant hat or hood
- Shoe covers
- Protective eyewear
- Disposable mask

Procedure

- Obtain a clean scrub top, pants, and a disposable hat or hood. Select a top and pants for proper fit and comfort.
- Remove jewelry, cracked or chipped nail polish, and street clothes.
- Cover hair with the bouffant hat or hood before donning the scrub top to prevent the possible dispersal of microorganisms and scalp hair onto the scrub attire.
- Adjust the hat or hood to cover all scalp hair. Persons with beards or long sideburns should obtain a beard cover to contain all facial hair.
- After donning the pants, tuck the top and pants' ties into the pants to prevent the possible dispersal of body scuff from beneath the shirt. Pants should not come in contact with the floor during dressing.
- Change to comfortable, supportive, protective footwear to protect the feet against falling items such as sharps and heavy instruments and to allow one to move quickly and safely in an emergency.
- Place disposable shoe covers over the shoes to protect footwear from gross contamination.
- On entering the restricted area of the surgical suite and other designated areas, such as the substerile area, the sterile center core, and the scrub sink area when team members are scrubbing, apply a surgical mask.
- Form the pliable nosepiece of the mask over the bridge of the nose; tie the mask at the back of the head and behind the neck, allowing the mask to fit securely and preventing venting at the sides. Change masks between procedures and remove them by handling the strings only.
- Avoid touching the filter portion of the mask and discard in an appropriate receptacle. Masks are either on or off; do not wear a mask around the neck, on top of the head, or in a pocket.
- Before scrubbing, apply protective eyewear or a mask with a protective splash guard visor to protect against uncontrolled body fluid splashes (OSHA Occupational exposure to bloodborne pathogens, 1991).
- During laser procedures, wear laser masks and protective eyewear specified for the type of laser in operation. Clean eyewear with an antimicrobial agent between surgical procedures.
- Do not wear surgical scrub attire outside the surgical suite. If laboratory coats or cover gowns are worn, they should have long sleeves, be completely closed, and fall below the knees.

Performing the Surgical Hand Scrub (AORN, 1992, *III*:8–1—8–5)

Supplies and Equipment

- Scrub sink with foot, knee, or automatic controls
- Water that is set at a comfortable temperature and moderate flow to prevent spraying of surgical attire
- High-filtration masks
- Scrub brushes
- Metal or plastic nail stick
- Broad spectrum antimicrobial agents (Table 1)

Procedure

- Inspect the OR attire by adjusting the hat or hood to cover and contain all hair. The mask should completely cover both the nose and the mouth and fit securely to prevent venting at the sides. Tuck all loose scrub attire and strings into the scrub pants. Replace or adjust shoe covers to completely protect shoes.
- Examine the hands and forearms for good skin integrity; remove all jewelry. Nails should be free from polish and short, and cuticles should be in good condition.
- Open the sterile scrub brush package and position it for easy access.
- Turn on the water, adjusting the temperature and spray so that scrub attire does not become wet.
- Wash and rinse the hands for the initial wash with water and a small amount of antimicrobial agent to remove transient flora and gross contaminants.
- Remove the plastic nail stick and the scrub brush from the package and add an antimicrobial agent from a dispenser or squeeze an impregnated sponge to generate lather. Clean nails and cuticles under running water with the plastic nail stick.
- Clean the nails and cuticles under running water while holding the scrub brush in the opposite hand; repeat for the other hand.
- Select either the anatomic timed scrub or the counted brush stroke method. Each takes about 5 minutes to complete.
- Anatomic timed scrub
  1. Scrub the nails for 30 seconds with brush.
  2. Scrub the fingers, including each side and web space, for 1 minute with sponge.
  3. Scrub palmar surfaces for 15 seconds with brush.
  4. Scrub dorsal surface 15 seconds with sponge.
  5. Scrub forearm, divided in half, to 2 inches above the elbow 1 minute with sponge (30 seconds each half).
  6. Repeat process for other hand.
- Counted brush stroke method

TABLE 1

Characteristics of Six Topical Antimicrobial Agents

Agent	Mode of Action	Rapidity of Action	Residual Activity	Usual Concentration (%)	Affected by Organic Matter
Alcohols	Denaturation of protein	Most rapid	None	70–92	No data
Chlorhexidine gluconate	Cell wall disruption	Intermediate	Excellent	4.2 in detergent base; 0.5 in alcohol	Minimal
Hexachlorophene	Cell wall disruption	Slow to intermediate	Excellent	3 by prescription only	Minimal
Iodine and iodophors	Oxidation/substitution by free iodine	Intermediate	Minimal	10, 7.5, 2, 0.5	Yes
Chloroxylenol	Cell wall disruption	Intermediate	Good	0.5–3.75	Minimal
Triclosan	Cell wall disruption	Intermediate	Excellent	0.3–1	Minimal

Adapted from Larson, E. (1988). APIC Guidelines for infection control practice, guideline for use of topical antimicrobial agents. *American Journal of Infection Control* 16: 253–266.

1. Scrub nails with 20 strokes with brush.
2. Scrub fingers, including each side and web space, 10 strokes with brush.
3. Scrub palmar surfaces 10 strokes with brush.
4. Scrub dorsal surface 10 strokes with sponge.
5. Scrub forearm, divided in half, to 2 inches above the elbow 40 strokes with sponge (10 strokes each side with sponge).
6. Repeat process for other hand.

- Beginning at the fingertips, scrub vigorously with vertical strokes, using the scrub brush. Proceed to the palm and the back of the hand. Scrub all four sides of each digit, including the web space.
- Proceed to the wrist; with a circular motion, continue up the forearm to 2 inches above the elbow.
- Scrub each anatomic area to ensure that all surfaces are sufficiently exposed to friction and an antimicrobial agent; repeat for other hand, and discard the scrub brush in an appropriate receptacle.
- Rinse the hands and arms thoroughly under running water, keeping the hands elevated to allow the water to drain off the flexed elbows.
- Take special care not to touch the faucet, clothing, or other objects and not to splash water onto the OR scrub attire. If the

Safety/Toxicity	Activity Against				
	Gram-Positive Bacteria	Gram-Negative Bacteria	Mycobacterium Tuberculosis	Fungi	Viruses
Drying, volatile	Excellent	Excellent	Good	Good	Good
Ototoxicity, keratitis	Excellent	Good	Poor	Fair	Good
Neurotoxicity	Excellent	Poor	Poor	Poor	Poor
Absorption from skin with possible toxicity, skin irritation	Excellent	Good	Good	Good	Good
More data needed	Good	Fair	Fair	Fair	Fair
More data needed	Good	Good except for Pseudomonas	Fair	Poor	Unknown

hands or forearms are touched, repeat the scrubbing procedure to correct the contamination.

- Proceed to the OR, with the hands held upward to allow water to drip off the elbows.

Donning Sterile Gown and Gloves (AORN, 1992, *III*:2–1)
Supplies and Equipment
- Sterile surgical gowns (wraparound style with sterile backs)
- Sterile absorbent towels
- Sterile disposable surgeon's gloves
- Separate sterile areas for the procedure are needed

Unassisted Gowning
SCRUB PERSON
- After completing the surgical hand scrub, grasp the folded towel near the corner with one hand and pull straight up. Pay careful attention not to drip water onto the sterile field.
- Step back from the sterile field, extend the arms, and lean slightly forward at the waist to prevent the towel from touching surgical attire.
- Unfold the towel, begin drying the hand with half the towel, and proceed to the wrist and forearm with a rotating motion, being careful not to retrace any surface.

- Grasp the untouched end of the towel with the dry hand and repeat the process on the other hand and forearm. Discard the towel in an appropriate receptacle.
- If the sterile towel touches the scrub attire, discard the contaminated towel and begin with another sterile towel.
- Grasp the folded gown at the neckline and step back from the sterile field, allowing the gown to unfold completely with the inside toward the wearer.
- Holding the arms at shoulder level, slide both arms simultaneously into the armholes.

CIRCULATING NURSE

- Assist the scrub person by reaching inside and pulling the gown up over the shoulders for proper sleeve adjustment. The cuffs are left extended over the hands for the closed glove technique, and the cuffs are pulled up to expose the hands for the assisted gloving technique.
- Tie the inside tie at the waist and secure the gown at the neckline. The final tie on a wraparound gown is completed after the sterile gloves have been donned.
- Complete closure on a sterile back gown in one of three ways:
  1. Grasp the belt tie and hand it to another sterile team member.
  2. For a disposable gown, hand the prepackaged card securing the belt tie to the circulating nurse.
  3. Secure the belt tie with an instrument and hand it off to the circulating nurse.
- Hold the prepackaged card or sterile instrument while the sterile team member pivots to the left, thereby completing the back closure of the gown. While retaining the cardboard or instrument, the scrub person pulls the belt tie free and ties the belts.

SCRUB PERSON

- Flex the arms at the elbows and hold them in front with both hands in sight at all times. Do not drop sterile hands below table or waist level.
- Consider gowns sterile in the front from shoulder to table level; sleeves are sterile from 2 inches above the elbow to the wrist, excluding the stockinet cuff.
- Consider the back of a wraparound unsterile because it cannot be observed by the scrubbed person (AORN, 1992, *III*:2–1).

Unassisted Gloving

CLOSED GLOVE TECHNIQUE

- While donning a sterile gown, slide the fingers into the sleeves until the cuff is reached.

- Open the inner glove wrapper on a sterile field. The gloves should be palm side up, with the glove labeled L on the left and that labeled R on the right (Fig. 1).
- Don the left glove first, turn the left hand palm side up, and flip the left glove onto the left palm. Place the folded glove cuff even with the gown cuff seam; the thumb of the glove is on the thumb side of hand and the fingers on the lunar side of the wrist, with the glove finger tips pointing toward the elbow (Fig. 2).

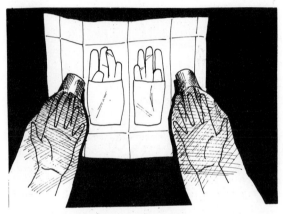

FIGURE 1   Open the glove wrapper on a sterile table.

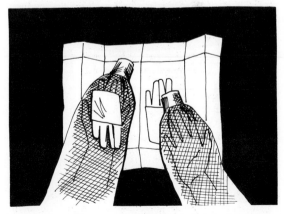

FIGURE 2   Place the left glove on the left palm.

- Grasp the lower edge of the glove cuff with the left thumb and index finger. Secure the upper edge of the glove cuff with the right thumb and index finger and stretch the entire glove cuff over the stockinet opening, being careful not to touch the edge of the stockinet cuff (Fig. 3).
- Work the fingers into the glove, then grasp the left glove and gown at the seam with the right hand and pull up over the wrist (Fig. 4).
- Turn the right hand palm side up, flip the right glove on the right palm. Place the folded glove cuff even with the gown cuff

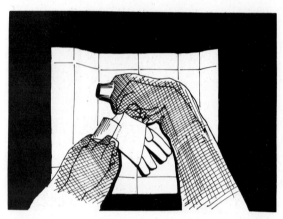

FIGURE 3   Grasp the left glove cuff.

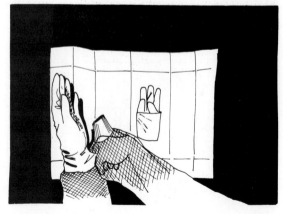

FIGURE 4   Pull the left glove up over the wrist.

seam; the thumb of the glove is on the thumb side of the hand and the fingers on the ulnar side of the wrist, with the glove finger tips pointing toward the elbow (Fig. 5).

- Grasp the lower edge of the glove cuff with the right thumb and index finger. Secure the upper edge of the glove cuff with the left thumb and index finger and stretch the entire glove cuff over the stockinet opening, being careful not to touch the edge of the stockinet cuff (Fig. 6).

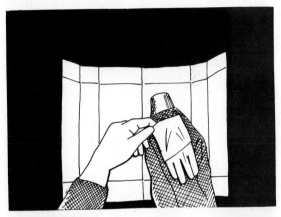

FIGURE 5   Place the right glove on the right palm.

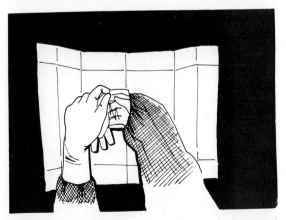

FIGURE 6   Stretch the entire right glove cuff over the stockinet opening.

- Work the fingers into the glove, then grasp the right glove and gown at the seam with the left hand and pull up over the wrist (Fig. 7).
- Adjust both gloves for comfort and fit (Fig. 8).
- Remove powder from gloves; its residue has been associated with the development of granulomas and peritonitis.

OPEN GLOVE TECHNIQUE
- Extend the hands through the sterile gown cuff.
- Ensure that exposed skin does not come in contact with the exterior of the sterile gloves.

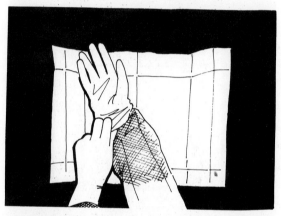

FIGURE 7 Pull the right glove up over the wrist.

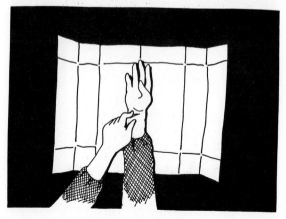

FIGURE 8 Adjust the gloves.

- Open the inner glove wrapper carefully to expose the gloves, making sure that the wrapper does not flip back and contaminate the gloves (Fig. 9).
- Grasp the right glove cuff on the fold with the left thumb and index finger, touching only the interior of the glove (Fig. 10).
- Insert the right hand into the glove and gently pull it on, leaving the cuff turned down (Fig. 11).
- Slide the fingers of the gloved right hand under the fold of the left cuff, touching only the exterior of the glove and insert the left hand (Fig. 12).

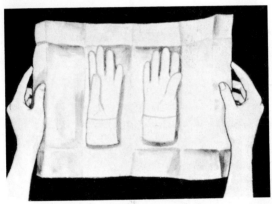

FIGURE 9 Open the glove wrapper. (Drawing provided by Baxter Pharmaseal.)

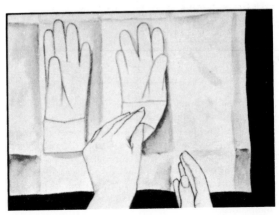

FIGURE 10 Grasp the right glove. (Drawing provided by Baxter Pharmaseal.)

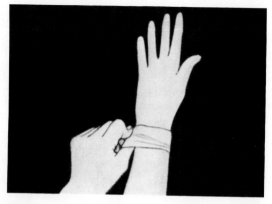

FIGURE 11 Pull on the right glove. (Drawing provided by Baxter Pharmaseal.)

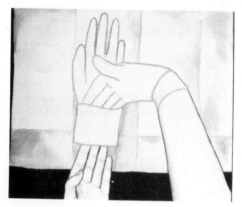

FIGURE 12 Slide the right fingers under the left glove cuff. (Drawing provided by Baxter Pharmaseal.)

- Gently pull it on and stretch the cuff over the stockinet cuff, avoiding inward rolling of the glove cuff (Fig. 13).
- Slide the fingers of the left gloved hand under the fold of the right cuff and stretch the glove cuff over the stockinet cuff, avoiding inward rolling of the glove cuff.
- Because the open glove technique provides a greater chance that the scrub person's hands come in contact with the sterile glove, thereby becoming contaminated, the closed glove method is recommended.

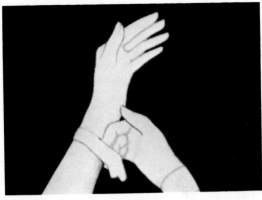

FIGURE 13   Pull on the left glove. (Drawing provided by Baxter Pharmaseal.)

Assisted Gowning

SCRUB PERSON

- Place an open sterile towel over the outstretched hand of the newly scrubbed team member.
- Pick up the gown at the neck, step back from the sterile field, and allow the gown to unfold completely.
- Form a protective cuff by placing the hands at shoulder level on the exterior side of the gown and drape the gown over the gloves.
- Identify the armholes and place the gown on the outstretched hands of the scrubbed team member.
- Release the gown.

CIRCULATING NURSE

- Assist the scrub person by reaching inside and pulling the gown up over the shoulder and securing it at the neck and at the waist with the inside tie.

Assisted Gloving

- Grasp the right glove under the inverted cuff (the right hand is usually gloved first in assisted gloving).
- Stretch the cuff while protecting the sterile thumbs and fingers by placing them under the cuff on the exterior side of the glove.
- Hold the stretched glove open, palm side toward the team member being gloved. Assist the team member's hand into the glove by gently pulling the glove upward as the team member pushes his or her hand into the glove.
- Cover the gown stockinet cuff completely with the sterile glove.
- Repeat the process for the other hand.

Regowning and Regloving

- When a glove becomes contaminated, there are three options for regloving:
  1. Ask for assistance from a sterile team member in regloving.
  2. Remove both gown and gloves and regown and reglove.
  3. Apply a sterile glove over the contaminated glove.

CIRCULATING NURSE

- To remove a contaminated glove, have the scrubbed person extend the glove out of the sterile field.
- While wearing protective gloves, pull off the contaminated glove, leaving the stockinet cuff in place.
- The closed glove technique cannot be used for regloving because the stockinet cuff is contaminated; therefore, ask a sterile team member to assist in gloving.
- If this is impossible, apply a sterile glove over the contaminated glove.
- When a gown becomes contaminated, untie the gown, then face the scrubbed team member and grasp the gown at the shoulders while inverting the gown as it is being taken off.
- Remove the gloves by touching the interior of the glove without touching the scrubbed hands of the sterile team member, turning the gloves inside out as they are removed.
- Don protective gloves before removing the gloves of the scrubbed person.
- The scrubbed team member is ready to regown and reglove.
- Contaminated gown and gloves are not to be worn outside the OR.

Preparing a Sterile Field (AORN, 1992, *III*:2–1—2–6)
Skin Preparation

SUPPLIES AND EQUIPMENT

- Shave preparation kit
- Nonsterile gloves
- Disposable or terminally sterilized reusable razor
- Skin solvents
- Antimicrobial detergent
- Depilatory cream
- Terminally sterilized electrical clippers and/or scissors
- Small separate movable table
- Sterile preparation tray, including bowls, or a plastic tray with compartments; sponges; sponge sticks; cotton-tipped applicators; sterile gloves
- Sterile absorbent towels
- Sterile nail cleaner
- Sterile brush

HAIR REMOVAL
- Check the patient care area for adequate lighting and patient privacy. Explain the procedure to the patient. Inquire about allergies, scars, or moles that may interfere with hair removal.

WET SHAVE
- Prepare towels, detergent, a sharp disposable or terminally sterilized razor, and a container with warm water.
- Expose the incisional area, and assess the patient's skin condition.
- Don nonsterile gloves and place an impervious towel beneath the area to be shaved.
- Lather the skin in the incisional area and let it set for a few minutes.
- Hold the skin taut and shave by moving the razor in the direction of hair growth, avoiding cutting or making nicks in the skin.
- Shave only the hair in the incisional area that interferes with the surgical procedure.
- After shaving, clean, rinse, and dry the skin and make the patient comfortable.

REMOVING HAIR WITH DEPILATORY CREAM
- A skin-sensitivity test should be performed before application. Apply the cream according to manufacturer's instructions.
- After the specified time, remove the cream and the hair.
- Clean, rinse, and dry the skin.

REMOVING HAIR WITH ELECTRICAL CLIPPERS OR SCISSORS
- Clip hair in the prescribed area to prevent contamination of the incisional area with hair.
- Trim long hair surrounding the incisional area so that it does not interfere with the surgical procedure.
- Document the patient's skin condition before and immediately after the hair removal, noting any redness, razor nicks, or skin abrasions.

Patient Skin Scrub

- Prepare sterile supplies for skin preparation on a separate, small movable table.
- Select broad-spectrum antimicrobial agents capable of reducing and inhibiting both transient and resident microorganisms (see Table 1).
- If unfamiliar with antimicrobial agent, read the manufacturer's instructions. Some can be neurotoxic, and some may be toxic or harmful at various body sites. Eye injury associated with chlorhexidine gluconate has been reported, and chlorhexidine gluconate can cause ototoxicity if instilled directly into the middle ear (Larson, 1988, p. 258).

- If the patient is awake, explain the procedure and provide privacy and comfort. Make every effort to allay fears, and answer questions in a reassuring manner.
- If the patient has been anesthetized, check with the anesthetist before starting the preparation.
- After the patient has been positioned, move the small table with the sterile skin prepping supplies close to the patient. Expose the area to be prepared, assessing the skin condition and the effectiveness of hair removal.
- Don sterile gloves and arrange supplies for the procedure. Since pooling of solutions may result in skin burn or irritation owing to chemical action, place absorbent towels on each side of the patient to absorb excess solution and to prevent pooling under the patient, electrodes, and the electrosurgical dispersive pad.
- To prevent pooling under tourniquets, seal off with an impervious U drape or towel. Also, place impervious pads under the extremities to prevent solutions from saturating the patient's linen.
- Begin cleansing at the incision site in a circular motion, moving out toward the periphery. When the edges of the preparation site have been reached, discard the used sponge and, with a new sterile sponge, repeat the process. Never bring a soiled sponge back toward the incisional site. Prepare at least 6 to 8 inches beyond the incisional site in all directions unless otherwise stated for a specific procedure (see below).
- Time the cleansing of the operative site to last long enough to thoroughly cleanse the skin.
- Use cotton-tipped applicators to thoroughly clean the umbilicus and hard-to-reach areas.
- Clean the preparation site from clean to dirty by scrubbing high-bioburden areas last and discarding the sponge. Areas of high bioburden are the umbilicus, the axillary area, the vagina, the anus, open skin lesions, soiled traumatic wounds, and stomas.
- If the incisional site includes a stoma as an integral part of the procedure, cover the stoma with a sterile gauze and cleanse the area surrounding the stoma; cleanse the stoma last. If the stoma is in the operative area, yet not included in the incision, isolate the stoma with a clear plastic adherent drape and then begin the preparation.
- Flush most open traumatic wounds, burns, or denuded areas with copious amounts of sterile solutions to flush contaminants out of the wound.
- Prepping after removal of a cast or large dressing may necessitate soaking with sterile solutions to remove adherent dressings. Exercise care in this situation because the skin may be sensitive and denuded.

- Prepping for procedures involving grafts necessitates separate setups; if the area is small, however, one preparation setup may be used. Clean the donor site first.
- When preparing an area with a possible malignancy (e.g., a breast mass), omit scrubbing to avoid the possible spread of carcinoma and only apply an antimicrobial paint or gel to the operative area.
- After scrubbing, wipe the lather off with a dry sponge or blot dry with an absorbent towel.
- When removing the towel, grasp the edges farthest away and lift the towel up away from the skin; the towel should be brought toward the person performing the preparation. Pay careful attention not to contaminate the prepared area with the edges of the towel.
- Use a sponge stick and an outward circular motion to apply the antimicrobial solution. Start at the incisional area and move to the periphery. Use a second and third sponge stick to completely cover the operative area.
- If flammable solutions are used (alcohol, acetone, fat solvents), ensure that adequate time elapses to allow the solution to dry and the fumes to evaporate before activating electrosurgical or laser equipment.
- Remove the impervious preparation pad from under the extremities or remove the absorbent towels from each side of the patient; avoid bringing towels over the prepared area.
- Remove the gloves and discard all preparation materials in a proper receptacle.
- Document on the OR record the patient's skin condition and the effectiveness of hair removal before beginning the preparation; state the antimicrobial agent used, the area prepared, and the person who performed the prep.
- On completion of the surgical procedure, assess the patient's skin in and around the operative site and document on the OR record any redness, abrasions, or burns. Communicate the findings to the surgeon and the postanesthesia care nurse.

Scrub for Specific Anatomic Areas

EYE (Fig. 14)
- Confine the patient's hair within a disposable surgical hat or towel.
- Secure the head in a head support to prevent rolling or moving.
- Trim the eyelashes (when ordered) with a fine scissors coated with sterile ophthalmic ointment to catch the lashes.
- Squeeze sponges almost dry when cleansing, to prevent pooling of the solution in the eye.

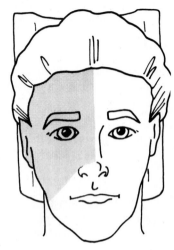

FIGURE 14 The shaded area is prepared for eye surgery.

- Cleanse the periorbital area, the eyelid, the lashes, and an area at least 1 inch in diameter beyond the periphery of the eye, using a nonirritating aqueous antimicrobial solution and sponges.
- Begin at the center of the eye and continue to the periphery, using cotton-tipped applicators for difficult-to-reach areas.
- Irrigate the periorbital area with a small bulb syringe and sterile water. Contain irrigating solution in a basin or with a towel at the side of the head.
- Blot the area dry with a sterile sponge.

LOWER FACE AND NOSE (Fig. 15)
- Confine the patient's hair within a disposable surgical hat or towel.
- Secure the head in a head support to prevent rolling or moving.
- Protect the patient's eyes with sponges or eye pads.
- Squeeze the sponges almost dry when cleansing to prevent pooling of the solution in the patient's eyes or ears.
- Begin cleansing at the bridge of the nose in a circular motion, moving out toward the hairline and down to the mandible.
- Use cotton-tipped applicators to cleanse the nostrils and hard-to-reach areas.
- Squeeze excess antimicrobial solution from the sponge stick and paint from the nose to the periphery.

EAR (Fig. 16)
- Confine the patient's hair within a disposable surgical hat or towel.

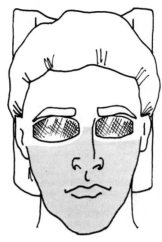

FIGURE 15 The shaded area is prepared for nose and lower face surgery.

- Turn the patient's head to the side, with the ear to be operated on up, and secure in a head support to prevent rolling or moving.
- When ordered, clip or wet-shave hair around the ear that may interfere with the procedure.
- Secure the patient's hair and define the operative area with tape or adhesive plastic towels.
- Squeeze the sponges almost dry when cleansing to prevent pooling of the solution in the ear.

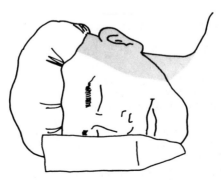

FIGURE 16 The shaded area is prepared for ear surgery.

- Prepare from the center of the ear, using a nonirritating antimicrobial solution. Extend the prep onto the face and neck area.
- Use cotton-tipped applicators to cleanse the external ear canal.
- A small piece of cotton ball may be placed in the external ear to absorb solution and prevent pooling of prepping solution.
- Squeeze excessive antimicrobial solution from the sponge stick and paint from the center of the ear. Extend the prep into the face and neck area.

NECK AND COMBINED HEAD AND NECK (Fig. 17)

- Expose the operative area to the nipple line.
- Place an impervious pad at the table line beneath the head.
- Begin cleansing in a circular motion from the incisional site to the periphery.
- Prepare the neck anteriorly and laterally from the mandible to midsternum, including the tops of the shoulders.
- For a combined head and neck procedure, also cleanse the lower portion of the face and the areas of the head around the ears.
- Continue the scrubbing long enough to cleanse the area thoroughly.
- Blot the area dry with absorbent sterile towels.
- Paint with an antimicrobial solution.

CHEST OR BREAST (Fig. 18)

- Support the fingers in a hand-holder device, or have an assistant elevate the patient's hand and arm.

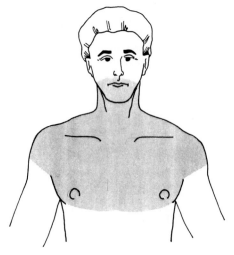

FIGURE 17 The shaded area is prepared for head and neck surgery.

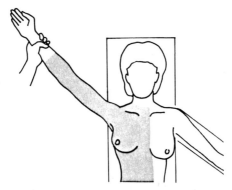

FIGURE 18   The shaded area is prepared for breast surgery.

- Expose the operative area to the waistline.
- Place an absorbent towel over the nonoperative side and an impervious preparation pad on the table under the axilla and shoulder of the operative side.
- Begin cleansing in a circular motion from the incisional site to the periphery.
- Prepare from the top of the shoulder to below the diaphragm and from the edge of the nonoperative breast to the table line, including the upper arm to elbow circumferentially and the axilla.
- Cleanse the axillary area last or use a separate sponge and discard it because of the high bioburden in that area.
- Prepare both sides of the chest for a bilateral procedure.
- Paint with an antimicrobial solution.
- For a breast biopsy, prepare the breast from the incisional area, to include an area approximately 3 inches in diameter beyond the breast.
- When preparing a breast with a possible malignancy, omit scrubbing to avoid possible spread of carcinoma; gently apply an antimicrobial paint or gel to the operative area only.

ABDOMEN, SUPINE POSITION (Fig. 19)

- Expose the operative area from the nipple line to the pubis.
- Place absorbent towels alongside the patient at the table line to absorb any solution and prevent pooling.
- Begin cleansing in a circular motion from the incisional site to the periphery.
- Prepare from the breast line to the groin area and from table line to table line.
- Continue scrubbing long enough to cleanse the area thoroughly.

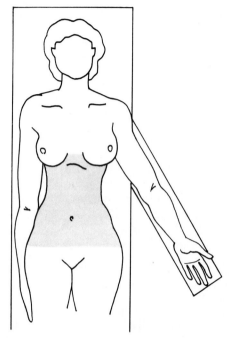

Figure 19 The shaded area is prepared for abdominal surgery.

- Blot the area dry with absorbent sterile towels.
- Paint with an antimicrobial solution.

BACK, PRONE POSITION (Fig. 20)

- Expose the operative area from the shoulders to the top of the buttocks.
- Place absorbent towels alongside the patient at the table line to absorb any solution and prevent pooling.
- Begin cleansing in a circular motion from the incisional site to the periphery.
- Prepare from the shoulders to the top of the buttocks and from table line to table line.
- Continue scrubbing long enough to cleanse the area thoroughly.
- Blot the area dry with absorbent sterile towels.
- Paint with an antimicrobial solution.

CHEST AND KIDNEY, LATERAL POSITION (Fig. 21)

- Expose the operative area to the ileum.
- Place absorbent towels anteriorly and posteriorly, under the chest at the table level.

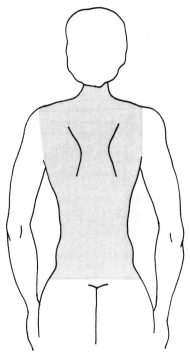

FIGURE 20   The shaded area is prepared for back surgery with the patient in the prone position.

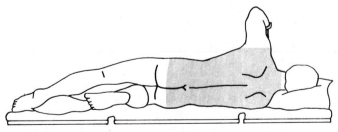

FIGURE 21   The shaded area is prepared for thoracic surgery with the patient in the lateral position.

- Begin cleansing in a circular motion from the incisional site to the periphery.
- Prepare the area from the shoulders to the ileum and the anterior and posterior chest wall for thoracic procedures.

- Prepare from midchest to the hip, anteriorly and posteriorly for kidney procedures.
- Blot the area dry with absorbent sterile towels.
- Paint with an antimicrobial solution.

PERINEUM OR VAGINA (Fig. 22)

- Expose the perineal area.
- Place an impervious pad under the buttocks and form a funnel into a kick bucket to collect fluids.
- Prepare from the pubis to the anus, including the vulva, the labia, the perineum, the inner aspects of the thighs, and the vagina.
- Cleanse from the pubis area downward over the vulva and the perineum and past the anus; always discard the sponge after touching the anus because of the high bioburden in that area.
- Scrub the inner aspects of the thighs, beginning at the labia majora and moving outward.
- Insert a narrow sponge stick saturated with an antimicrobial agent gently into the vagina and, using a rotating motion, cleanse the many folds of the vaginal mucosa. Repeat twice, discarding the sponge stick after each use.
- Insert a dry narrow sponge gently into the vagina to absorb any pooling of antimicrobial agent.

CATHETERIZATION IN CONJUNCTION WITH PERINEAL-VAGINAL PREPARATION

- Remove the gloves; they are considered contaminated from the preparation.
- Don sterile gloves and insert a sterile catheter.

HAND OR FOREARM (Fig. 23)

- Apply a tourniquet to the upper arm, when ordered (see Chapter 8).

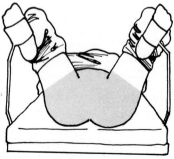

FIGURE 22 The shaded area is prepared for perineal or vaginal surgery.

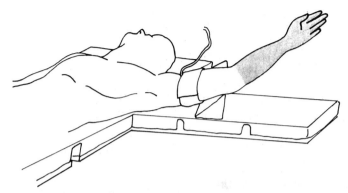

FIGURE 23 The shaded area is prepared for hand or forearm surgery.

- Place the patient's arm on a hand table, which is protected with an impervious pad.
- Elevate the forearm on an extremity support.
- Begin cleansing at the fingertips and continue to the elbow circumferentially, paying close attention to areas under the nails and the cuticles.
- If the nail beds are dirty, soak a sudsy solution under the nails and clean with a nail cleaner and brush.
- Blot the area dry with absorbent sterile towels.
- Paint with an antimicrobial solution from the fingertips to the elbow.

ELBOW AND UPPER ARM (Fig. 24)

- Apply a tourniquet to the upper arm, when ordered (see Chapter 8).
- Support the fingers in a hand-holder device or have an assistant elevate the patient's hand and arm.
- Apply an impervious adhesive U drape, sealing off a tourniquet to prevent the preparation solution from running or pooling under the tourniquet.
- Begin cleansing in a circular motion from the incisional site to the periphery.
- Prepare from the wrist to the axilla or to the tourniquet, if one has been applied, circumferentially.
- Continue the scrubbing long enough to cleanse the area thoroughly.
- Blot the area dry with absorbent sterile towels.
- Paint with an antimicrobial solution from the incisional site to the periphery.

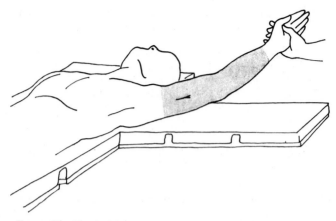

FIGURE 24   The shaded area is prepared for elbow and upper arm surgery.

SHOULDER (Fig. 25)
- Support the fingers in a hand-holder device or have an assistant elevate the patient's shoulder from the table.
- Place an impervious pad under the shoulder and axilla.
- Begin cleansing in a circular motion from the incisional site to the periphery.

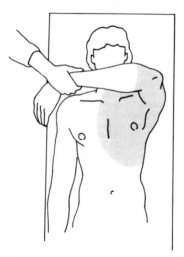

FIGURE 25   The shaded area is prepared for shoulder surgery.

- Prepare from midneck to the elbow circumferentially, including the shoulder, the scapula, the chest to the nipple, and the axilla.
- Cleanse the axillary area last, or use a separate sponge and discard because of the high bioburden in that area.
- Continue scrubbing long enough to cleanse the area thoroughly.
- Blot the area dry with absorbent sterile towels.
- Paint with an antimicrobial solution from the incisional site to the periphery.

HIP, SEMILATERAL POSITION (Fig. 26)

- Support the foot in an extremity-holder device or have an assistant elevate the patient's entire leg from the groin to the ankle.
- Apply an impervious adhesive U drape, isolating the perineal-rectal area.
- Begin cleansing in a circular motion from the incisional site to the periphery.
- Prepare from the waist to midbuttocks and to the lower outer aspect of the abdomen; include the leg circumferentially from the hip to the ankle.
- Blot the area dry with absorbent sterile towels.
- Paint with an antimicrobial solution from the incisional site to the periphery.

HIP, FRACTURE TABLE (Fig. 27)

- Position the patient on a fracture table with the affected leg in traction.
- Apply an impervious adhesive U drape, isolating the perineal-rectal area.
- Place an impervious pad between the affected hip and the top of the fracture table.

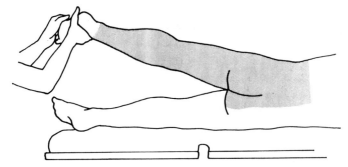

FIGURE 26 The shaded area is prepared for hip procedures with the patient in the semilateral position.

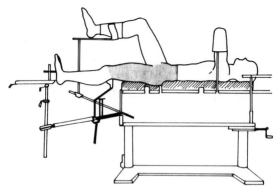

FIGURE 27 The shaded area is prepared for hip procedures with the patient on the fracture table.

- Begin cleansing in a circular motion from the incisional site to the periphery.
- Prepare from the waist to the abdominal midline and to the table level and include the leg circumferentially from the hip to the knee.
- Continue scrubbing long enough to cleanse the area thoroughly.
- Blot the area dry with absorbent sterile towels.
- Paint with an antimicrobial solution from the incisional site to the periphery.

KNEE (Fig. 28)

- Support the foot in an extremity-holder device or have an assistant elevate the entire leg from the table.
- Apply a tourniquet to the upper thigh, when ordered (see Chapter 8).
- Apply an impervious U drape, sealing off the tourniquet to prevent the solution from running or pooling under the tourniquet.
- Prepare circumferentially from the ankle to the tourniquet.
- Begin cleansing at the knee in a circular motion, moving up toward the tourniquet, and discard sponges.
- Begin cleansing again at the knee in a circular motion to the ankle and discard sponges.
- Continue scrubbing long enough to cleanse the area thoroughly.
- Blot the area dry with absorbent sterile towels.
- Paint with an antimicrobial agent from the knee to the tourniquet and discard the paint stick. With another paint stick, paint from the knee to the ankle.

FOOT OR ANKLE (Fig. 29)

- Apply a tourniquet to the upper thigh, when ordered (see Chapter 8).

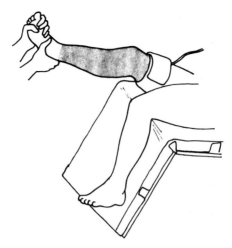

FIGURE 28 The shaded area is prepared for knee procedures.

- Elevate the lower leg on an extremity support.
- Place an impervious pad under the foot.
- Begin cleansing at the toes and move up toward the lower leg.
- Prepare from the tip of the toes to the midcalf circumferentially, paying close attention to the area under and around the nails.
- Blot the area dry with absorbent sterile towels.
- Paint with an antimicrobial solution, starting at the toes and moving up toward the calf.

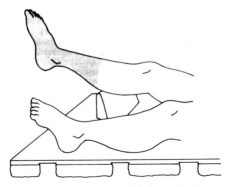

FIGURE 29 The shaded area is prepared for foot and ankle procedures.

OPEN HEART (Fig. 30)

- Expose the operative area from the neck to the toes.
- Elevate the legs on an ankle support.
- Place an impervious pad under the legs and towels alongside the patient at the table line to absorb excessive solution.
- Prepare from the trachea to the toes, including both legs circumferentially.
- Begin cleansing in a circular motion at the sternum and move toward the periphery of the torso.
- Prepare the leg circumferentially, beginning at the incision area, to the periphery of the legs.
- Prepare the genital area separately and isolate the area with an impervious towel.
- Continue scrubbing long enough to cleanse the area thoroughly.
- Blot the area dry with absorbent sterile towels.
- Paint with an antimicrobial solution from the incisional site to the periphery.
- Separate preps may be done for the chest area and the leg areas.

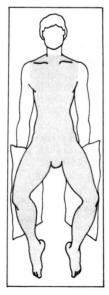

FIGURE 30 The shaded area is prepared for open heart surgery.

Draping the Patient and Equipment (AORN, 1992, *III*:2–1 and 6–1)

Considerations (Table 2)

Supplies and Equipment

- Barrier drapes
- Fenestrated sheets
- Drape sheets (three-quarter sheets, half-sheet, medium sheet)
- Impervious table covers
- Incise drape
- U drape
- Towel drape
- Aperture drape
- Isolation drape

TABLE **2**

Principles of Draping

1. Aseptically prepare the operative site before applying sterile surgical drapes.
2. Impervious fluid-proof drapes provide an effective sterile barrier and must be used when soaking of blood and body fluids is a potential risk.
3. Fluid-resistant drapes provide an effective sterile barrier when splashing and spraying of body fluids is a potential risk.
4. Sterile drapes should be handled as little as possible; avoid shaking, fanning, or haphazard unfolding.
5. Drapes are carried folded to the operative site and are considered nonsterile if allowed to fall below the waist or table level.
6. The area around the incision is draped first and then the periphery.
7. When placing drapes, never reach across the nonsterile area to drape the other side; go around; all draping is done from the appropriate side.
8. Form a cuff with the sterile drape to protect the sterile gloved hands when draping the periphery or equipment.
9. Hold the drapes high enough to avoid touching the nonsterile areas of the OR bed.
10. After a drape is placed, it is not moved or repositioned. Drapes that are incorrectly placed or become contaminated are removed by the circulating nurse, with care not to contaminate the operative site or other drapes.
11. A towel clip that has been placed through a drape has contaminated points and must not be repositioned or removed until completion of the procedure.
12. If the sterility of a drape is questionable, discard it.

Data from Atkinson, L. J., Kohn, M. L. (1986). *Berry and Kohn's introduction to operating room technique* (6th ed) (pp. 317–318). New York: McGraw-Hill Book Co. Kneedler, J. A., Dodge, G. H. (1987). *Perioperative patient care* (2nd ed) (pp. 454–456). Boston: Blackwell Scientific Publications. Groah, L. (1983). *Operating room nursing: The perioperative role*. Reston, Va: Reston Publishing Co.

- Stockinet
- Equipment drapes

Draping Equipment

- Inspect the area in the OR where the sterile field will be set up.
- Assemble furniture and equipment to be draped within the sterile field.
- Check the surfaces of tables and equipment for cleanliness and dryness.
- Gather all necessary draping supplies for the proposed surgery.
- Inspect the outer package for holes. If the integrity of the package has not been compromised, it is ready for use. If there are any defects, discard it.
- Use fluid-proof barrier drapes with impervious backing for sterile barriers for back tables and Mayo stands.

Draping of the Back Table by a Nonsterile Team Member

- Remove the drape pack from the outer package.
- Place the drape pack on the center of the back table.
- Tear the seal and open toward the back of the table first and then open toward the front of the table. A nonsterile person should open the flap farthest away from her or him first and the nearest flap last.
- Walk to either end of the table and grasp the cuff below table level and unfold the back table cover toward yourself. Move to the other side of the table and repeat the same movements. The area touched falls below the nonsterile table level, leaving the surface of the table sterile while exposing the pack contents.

Draping of the Back Table by Sterile Team Members

- Open the table drape toward yourself to cover the nonsterile front edge of the table first to minimize the possibility of contaminating the front of the gown.
- Protect gloved hands in the folded cuffs and place a drape over the back of the table and then laterally to each side.

Draping of the Mayo Stand by a Sterile Team Member

- Place both hands under the cuff, palms down. A Mayo stand cover is a long tube (pillowcase-like) drape.
- Slide the cover over the Mayo stand, allowing it to unfold as it is being applied and taking precautions not to let it fall below waist level.
- Stabilize the Mayo stand by placing a foot on its base while sliding the cover on.
- Adjust the lower open end of the Mayo stand cover by pulling the cuff down the stand. This is done by a nonsterile team member.

- Arrange all drapes in sequence of their use and handle the drapes as little as possible.

Draping for Specific Procedures and Anatomic Areas

LAPAROTOMY OR ANY FLAT SURFACE

- Hand sterile adhesive drape towels, with the folded adhesive edge toward yourself, to the surgeon or place the adhesive towel, folded edge toward the patient, to outline the operative site.
- If linen huck towels are used, fold one third of the towel lengthwise with the folded side toward yourself and hand it to the surgeon or place the folded edge toward the patient to outline the operative site.
- Remove the release liners from the adhesive strips around the fenestration; place the folded laparotomy sheet with the fenestration directly over the operative site.
- Unfold the drape to each side, keeping it at table level until it is unfolded toward the patient's head, including arm boards, and toward the patient's feet, including an adequate length over the OR bed.

EYE, EAR, NOSE, AND FACE

- Place the gloved hands, palms down, under the cuff of the head or bar drape.
- Place the head or bar drape under the patient's head while a nonsterile team member lifts up the patient's head.
- Remove the release liner tabs from adhesive strips and draw the drape up separately on each side of the patient's face (turban style) and secure with adhesive.
- Place a split sheet on the patient's chest with the tails toward the head, unfold to the sides and then to the feet. Remove release liners from adhesive strips and simultaneously position the tails while adhering them around the operative site.
- Apply a small-aperture drape by removing the release liner from the adhesive and then securing the edges to the skin around the operative site.
- When applying drapes around the head and face of an awake patient, provide adequate breathing space and protect the patient from fear of claustrophobia.

LITHOTOMY

SEPARATE LEGGINGS AND SHEET

- Place the gloved hands, palms up, under the cuff of the underbuttocks drape and position it under the patient's buttocks.
- Protect the gloved hands in the legging cuff and apply the legging over the leg and the stirrup. The telescope fold allows for ease of positioning. Repeat for the other leg.
- Place the sheet on the abdomen (firmly pressing the adhesive strip to stabilize the drape) and unfold laterally; then unfold to the head.

ONE-PIECE DRAPE WITH ATTACHED LEGGINGS

- Remove the release liner from the adhesive strip.
- Place the fenestration over the perineal area.
- Unfold the drape toward the patient's head while firmly pressing the adhesive strip to the patient's abdomen to stabilize the drape.
- Grasp the legging marked "toe" with the right hand and pull it up over the patient's right leg and stirrup.
- Touching only the underside of the drape, the nonsterile team member assists in placing the drape over the patient's leg and stirrup.
- Repeat with the left hand for the left leg.
- Some drapes are designed with plastic pouches to help contain and control blood and body fluids.

HAND

- Drape the hand table with an impervious fluid-proof table cover.
- Apply a rolled towel around the arm and secure it with a clip. If stockinet is preferred, the towel may be omitted.
- Position the hand drape over the hand; grasp and pull the patient's hand through the elastic fenestration. Unfold the drape onto the hand table and across the patient's chest. Unfold toward the patient's feet, and unfold to the patient's head.

SHOULDER

- With the patient's arm and shoulder elevated, apply a U drape by removing the release liners from the adhesive strips and securing them to the skin below the arm, sealing off the axillary area.
- Apply an impervious stockinet if the arm is draped within the sterile field. Twist it to achieve a better fit and to expel the air as it is rolled up the arm.
- Apply an incise drape around the support apparatus if the arm is in traction.
- Position the body split sheet below the arm at the axilla; unfold the sheet side to side, then toward the patient's feet. Fold back the tails and remove the release liner from the adhesive strips.
- Seal the adhesive tails around the shoulder and toward the patient's head.
- Position the shoulder drape with the pouch above the shoulder. The arrow points toward the patient's feet. Unfold the drape from side to side and up to create the anesthesia screen.
- Unfold the tails toward the anesthesia screen to expose the incise release liner, remove the release liner, bring both tails down around the shoulder simultaneously, and seal the adhesive to the bottom split sheet.

HIP, SEMILATERAL POSITION

- With the patient's leg elevated, apply a U drape by removing the release liner from the adhesive strips and securing them to the skin, sealing off the perineal area and crossing the tails up over the iliac crest to complete the fenestration.

- Apply an impervious stockinet, twisting it to achieve a better fit and to expel the air as it is rolled up the leg.
- Position the split sheet under the leg, with the tails toward the operative site. Unfold the drape to each side and then to the feet.
- Fold back the tails and remove the release liners from the adhesive strips and simultaneously position the tails, adhering them around the operative site.
- Position the top sheet with the arrow toward the incision, unfold to the side, remove the release liners from the adhesive strip, and seal to the split sheet, completing the fenestration around the operative site. Unfold upward to create the anesthesia screen.
- If an elastic fenestrated hip sheet is used, follow steps 1 and 2. Slip the fenestration over the patient's foot and unfold to each side and then toward the foot and upward to create the anesthesia screen.
- If an incise drape is used, apply it over the operative site, securing the stockinet and all drapes in place.

HIP, FRACTURE TABLE
- Square off the operative site with adhesive drape towels.
- Apply an isolation hanging drape by removing the release liner from the incise area of the drape and firmly pressing the adhesive onto the operative site to stabilize the drape.
- Unfold laterally to each side. Unfold to top toward the support bar.
- Touching only the underside of the drape, the nonsterile team member assists in adhering the wall drape to the support bar.
- Unfold toward the floor.

ARTHROSCOPY
- With the patient's leg elevated, apply a U drape by removing the release liner from the adhesive strips and securing them to the leg above the knee, sealing off the tourniquet and the leg-holder device.
- Apply an impervious stockinet, twisting it to achieve a better fit and to expel the air as it is rolled up the leg.
- Position the arthroscopy drape with the fluid control pouch at the knee. Grasp the foot and pull the patient's leg through the double elastic fenestrations with the pouch.
- Unfold the drape to each side, then to the head and to the feet.
- To form a pouch, place one elastic fenestration above the knee and the other below the knee.
- If an elastic fenestrated arthroscopy drape is used without a pouch, follow steps 1 and 2.
- Slip the fenestration over the patient's foot and unfold to each side and then to the head and to the feet.

ANKLE OR FOOT
- With the patient's foot elevated, place an impervious fluid-proof barrier drape under the operative extremity.
- Apply a rolled towel around the patient's thigh and secure it with a clip. If stockinet is preferred, the towel may be omitted.
- Position the elastic fenestrated extremity sheet over the foot. Grasp and pull the patient's foot through the elastic fenestration.
- Unfold the drape to each side, then to the head and to the foot.

OPEN HEART
- With the patient's legs elevated, place an impervious fluid-proof barrier drape under the legs.
- Place stockinet on each foot or drape the feet in a small drape. Lower the patient's legs onto the sterile barrier.
- Seal off the perineal area with an impervious towel or drape.
- Apply adhesive drape towels along the sides of the patient's chest and legs.
- Apply a large incise sheet to cover the chest and the abdomen.
- Apply a large incise sheet over both legs and the groin area.
- Position a cardiovascular split drape on the patient's chest; remove the release liners from the adhesive and secure to the patient's chest.

PERFORMING SPONGE, SHARPS, AND INSTRUMENT COUNTS

The perioperative nurse demonstrates competency to perform sponge, sharps, and instrument counts by
- Following OR policy and procedure for counting
- Initiating incorrect count procedures
- Documenting the count results according to OR policy and procedure (AORN, 1992)

Counting Sponges

- Count sponges before the beginning of the procedure, when there is a change of personnel, when sponges are added to the sterile field, before the closure of a deep or large incision or body cavity, and immediately before completion of the procedure.
- As the circulating nurse, count sponges out loud with the scrub person.
- As the scrub person, separate the sponges when counting. This enables the circulating nurse to verify that additional sponges, or pieces of sponge, are not concealed.
- Use only x-ray–detectable sponges during the procedure.
- Count sponges in units of 5 or 10, depending on how they are packaged.

- Remove packages of sponges that contain more or less than the packaged number from the operative field.
- Do not remove counted sponges from the OR during the procedure.
- As the scrub person, keep sponges organized at all times on the operative field.
- Discard used sponges in an fluid-impervious, lined container.
- Count and bag sponges in groups of 5 or 10 as they are accumulated. After bagging sponges, label the bag with the number of sponges contained in the bag and initial.

Counting Sharps

- Count sharps before the beginning of the procedure, when there is a change of personnel, when sharps are added to the sterile field, before the closure of a deep or large incision or body cavity, and immediately before completion of the procedure.
- As the circulating nurse, count sharps aloud with the scrub person.
- Count needles according to the number indicated on the package. When the package is opened, the circulating nurse verifies the number of needles with the scrub person.
- Do not remove counted sharps from the OR during the procedure.
- Use sharps-counting devices to assist in the counting procedure.
- As the scrub person, keep sharps organized at all times on the operative field.
- As the scrub person, continually count needles during the procedure and hand them to the surgeon on an exchange basis.
- Account for all pieces of broken sharps.

Counting Instruments

- Count instruments before the beginning of the procedure, when there is a change of personnel, when instruments are added to the sterile field, before the closure of a deep or large incision or body cavity, and immediately before completion of the procedure.
- As the circulating nurse, count instruments aloud with the scrub person.
- Use uniform instrument sets. This allows easy identification and counting.
- Use preprinted instrument work sheets. The work sheet should match each instrument set.
- Do not remove counted instruments from the OR during the procedure.

- As the scrub person, keep the instruments organized at all times on the operative field.
- Account for all pieces of broken instrument.

Incorrect Counts

- In the event of an incorrect count, notify the surgeon and re-count.
- If the problem is still not resolved after a recount, search for the missing item. Ask the surgeon to explore the wound. Look in areas where the item could be concealed, such as under the OR bed, under the surgeon's or an assistant's feet, under instrument trays, and in trash containers.
- Request an x-ray film before the patient is taken from the OR.
- Implement documentation procedures according to policy and procedure.

Documentation and Communication Procedures

- As the circulating nurse or the scrub person, maintain communication about the status of sponge, sharps, and instrument counts throughout the procedure.
- As the circulating nurse, announce the results of the count to the surgeon. The surgeon should acknowledge the results of the count.
- Document the results of the count in the patient's record in compliance with facility's policy and procedure. Documentation includes
  1. Types and number of counts taken
  2. Names and titles of personnel taking the counts
  3. Results of counts
  4. Actions taken if discrepancies occur
  5. Rationale if counts are not performed or completed
  6. Signature of the responsible party (AORN, 1992)

PROVIDING INSTRUMENTS, EQUIPMENT, AND SUPPLIES

The perioperative nurse demonstrates competency to provide instruments, equipment, and supplies by safely and efficiently

- Selecting instruments, equipment, supplies, and suture for a surgical procedure
- Delivering instruments, supplies, and suture to the sterile field
- Arranging instruments and supplies on the instrument table and the Mayo tray
- Passing instruments and supplies to the surgeon
- Preparing and passing sutures to the surgeon
- Applying and removing a pneumatic tourniquet

- Applying and removing the electrosurgical unit dispersive electrode
- Operating the electrosurgical unit generator
- Preparing electrical instruments for use
- Preparing air-powered instruments for use
- Preparing the hyperthermia or hypothermia unit for use
- Applying dressings
- Assisting with the application of casts and splints

Selecting Instruments, Equipment, Supplies, and Suture for a Surgical Procedure

- Obtain the surgeon's preference card, pick list, and other forms used to select instruments, equipment, and supplies.
- Select all items listed on the surgeon's preference card and other pertinent forms. Make a list of the items not available.
- Check all sterile items for signs of moisture, lack of seal integrity, and compromise of packaging material, such as pinholes and tears.
- Note the expiration dates. If a discrepancy is found, do not use the item.
- Examine the autoclave tape on cloth-wrapped packages and the chemical sterilization indicators on or in paper or plastic packages for a color change to ensure that the item was subjected to a sterilization cycle. If a discrepancy is found, do not use the item.
- If the setup is not immediately used, return the surgeon's preference card to the appropriate location.
- Close the case cart or cover the setup with a cloth sheet or other appropriate protective material and label with the surgeon's name, the date and time of the procedure, and the procedure name.
- Establish accountability by initialing the label and place the setup in the appropriate location.
- If items are missing from the setup, make a list of missing items and attach it to the setup. Communicate the list of missing items to the appropriate person.

Delivering Instruments, Supplies, and Suture to the Sterile Field
General Guidelines

- Check all sterile items for signs of moisture, lack of seal integrity, compromise of packaging material, outdated expiration dates, and the absence of autoclave tape and chemical sterilization indicators of a color change before opening. If a discrepancy is found, do not use the item.
- Do not reach over the sterile field when delivering sterile items.

- Do not use cloth-wrapped items that are dropped on the floor. The decision to open the inner wrappers or packages of double-wrapped or double-packaged items is determined by institutional policy (*AORN Journal*, 1990, p. 440; U.S. Army, 1988, p. 35).

Wrapped Items

- Remove the autoclave tape and position the package so that it can be opened by lifting the top flap away from the body.
- Lift the top flap (first flap) away from the body, the second and third flaps to the left and the right, and the last flap toward the body.
- Gather the wrapper tails together with one hand when presenting the item to the sterile field.
- Open the wrappers for sharp, bulky, or heavy items on an appropriate-sized table or a Mayo stand (U.S. Army, 1988, pp. 47–48).

Items Sealed in Peel-Back Packages

- Carefully peel the package apart and present the item to the scrub person.
- The scrub person grasps the item and carefully lifts it from the package. The item must not touch the package's inner seal line during removal.
- If the scrub person cannot accept the sterile item, flip the item onto the sterile field. The item must not touch the inner seal line while being passed to the sterile field (U.S. Army, 1988, pp. 47–48).

Arranging Instruments and Supplies on the Instrument Table and Mayo Tray
General Guidelines

- Divide back table into four sections.
- The scrub person stands next to the left and right lower sections.
- If instruments are numerous, use a second back table or a Mayo stand and tray.
- Facilitate the continuity of care during staff changes by uniformly setting up back tables and Mayo trays.
- Before transferring an instrument set or other items to the back table, check the internal chemical sterilization indicator for a color change.
- If the color of the indicator has not changed or if the indicator is missing, remove the item and regown and reglove.

Examples of Surgical Instruments (Table 3)
Setting Up the Back Table

- Place the instrument pan with instruments in the far upper right quadrant of the back table.

- Prepare towels for use on the Mayo tray and the back table by completely rolling two towels into cylinders.
- Place one towel lengthwise and next to the edge of the Mayo tray.
- Place the other towel in the far lower right quadrant of the back table.
- Lift the stringed instruments from the instrument pan, place them on the rolled towel, and remove the stringer.
- Arrange the retractors according to size in the upper right quadrant, to the left of the instrument pan.
- If preferred, leave retractors in the instrument pan and arrange according to size.
- Arrange tissue and dressing forceps in the lower right quadrant of the back table, to the left of the rolled towel.
- Place scissors in the left front quadrant of the back table, next to the tissue and dressing forceps.
- Place suture packages and free needles in the left front quadrant of the back table, to the left of the scissors.
- Place needle holders in the left front quadrant of the back table, to the left of the suture packages and free needles.
- Close the box locks of the small and large towel clips and place them on the ring stand.
- Arrange sponges, special instruments, and supplies in the upper left quadrant of the back table.
- Place the irrigation bowl or pitcher in the upper left quadrant.

Preparing Scalpels
- Hold the scalpel handle in nondominant hand.
- With the dominant hand, grasp the blade on the dull edge with a needle holder at the widest, strongest point without touching the cutting edge.
- Point the blade and handle down and away from the body; slide the blade into the groove of the scalpel handle until it is secured.
- Place assembled scalpels ready for use on the back instrument table.

Setting Up the Mayo Tray
- Arrange suture ties on the covered Mayo tray and draped Mayo stand.
- Place silk and other nonabsorbable ties to the rear, away from the scrub person.
- Place absorbable ties to the front.
- Drape a towel over the ties and tuck under the tray.
- Arrange the clamps and hemostats needed for the first phase of the procedure on the rolled towel.
- Place the tissue forceps and scissors next to the instruments.

TABLE 3
Examples of Surgical Instruments

Category	Name
Grasping or holding clamps	Mosquito
	Crile
	Kelly
	Allis
	Babcock
	Right angle
	Kocher-Oscher
	Rochester-Péan
	Sponge forceps
	Tissue
	Dressing
	Adson
Needle holders	Hegar-Mayo
	Collier
	Brown
Retractors	Richardson (large and small)
	Army-Navy
	Vein
	Volkmann (sharp and dull)
Suction devices	Poole
	Yankauer tonsil
Scissors	Straight Mayo
	Curved Mayo
	Metzenbaum
Scalpels	Knife handle No. 4
	Knife handle No. 3
	Knife handle No. 7

Adapted from U.S. Army. (1988). 301-91D10 *Operating room specialist course competency based program of instruction student handbook.* Fort Sam Houston, Tex.: Academy of Health Sciences, U.S. Army.

- Place the scalpels next to the tissue forceps and scissors. The blade should point away from the scrub person.
- Place four sponges, suction tubing, the electrosurgical unit active electrode, the electrode holster with attachment hardware, and light handles or gloves on the Mayo tray.
- If the suction or active electrode tubing is attached to the drapes with a nonpenetrating clamp, insert the tubing or the cord through the handle rings of the clamp.

Uses
Control superficial bleeders and handle delicate tissue
Control bleeders in subcutaneous tissue
Control bleeders in muscle tissue; hold Kitner forceps; pass drains
Retract tissue; grasp fascia, cysts, and knee cartilage
Grasp appendix, fallopian tubes, ureters, intestines, and stomach
Pull suture strands around or behind vessels; perform dissection; clamp deep bleeders in hard-to-reach places
Grasp fascia on large patients when placing retention suture; grasp bone and cartilage; grasp uterine broad ligaments
Secure Kitner forceps; grasp broad ligaments of uterus; cross-clamp intestines
Secure sponges; extract placenta from uterus; grasp tough tissue
Grasp and hold fascia and subcutaneous tissue
Hold gauze sponges and dressings; grasp and hold delicate tissue
Perform skin closure
Hold medium- to heavy-gauge needles
Hold medium-gauge needles
Hold small-gauge needles
Retract broad tissue such as subcutaneous tissue
Use for shallow incisions and tissue
Use for shallow areas in arms and legs and veins
Use for shallow incisions during orthopedic surgery
Abdominal cavity and obstetric and gynecologic surgery
Use for a wide variety of surgical procedures
Cut suture and other surgical materials such as dressings and drains
Cut heavy, tough tissue such as muscle, fascia, and subcutaneous tissue; perform gross dissection
Cut delicate tissue such as peritoneum, intestines, and stomach; perform delicate dissection
Fits blade No. 20; use for skin knife
Fits blades Nos. 10, 11, 12, and 15; use for second knife
Fits blades Nos. 10, 11, 12, and 15; use for eye, hand, and plastic surgery

- Attach the Yankauer tonsil suction tip to the tubing and the electrode tip to the pencil.

Passing Instruments and Supplies to the Surgeon

- Pass the scalpel to the surgeon handle first with the cutting edge pointed downward.
- Pass tissue forceps and ringed or box-locked instruments in the position of function.

- Assemble multipiece retractors before passing to the surgeon.
- Pass retractors handle first.
- Place sponges close to the operative site. Moisten and wring out sponges as requested by the surgeon. Sponges for the abdominal or thoracic cavity are usually moistened.
- Pass Kittner dissector sponges held in a Kelly clamp or Rochester-Péan forceps and stick sponges on a sponge forceps.
- Pass instruments by gently snapping them into the surgeon's hand. Release the instrument as soon as the surgeon has a firm grip.

Preparing and Passing Suture to the Surgeon
Nonabsorbable Suture

- Tear the foil pack at the notch and remove the suture strands from the package as a unit.
- Unfold the strands of suture to full length.
- Do not pull silk suture between gloved fingers. This prevents the buildup of static electricity in the suture.
- Place the strands under the towel on the Mayo tray according to type and size.

Absorbable Suture

- Tear the foil pack over a small basin to prevent fluid from dripping on the table drape.
- Remove the suture from the package.
- Place the center loop of the suture over two fingers of the nondominant hand and unwind the suture to half-length.
- Gently pull to straighten the suture. Jerking the strand can lead to breakage.
- Fold and cut the suture into equal parts and cut with the suture scissors.
- Place the strands under the towel on the Mayo tray according to type and size.

Preparing Free Ties

- Hold both ends of the suture securely with one end in each hand.
- Press the tie firmly into the palm of the surgeon's dominant hand.
- Release the suture as soon as the surgeon closes his or her hand.

Preparing Tie-to-Pass Ligatures

- Place the tip of the suture strand securely into the tip of a tonsil or right-angled clamp and lock the clamp.
- Hold the box lock of the clamp between the thumb and the index finger.

- The tip of the clamp should be positioned so that it faces the back of the hand.
- Gently snap the rings of the clamp into the palm of the surgeon's hand so that the tip of the clamp points toward the center of the surgeon's body.

Preparing Stick-Tie Sutures

- Position the needle in the needle holder so that the point of the needle faces the midline and the suture end of the needle is on the right.
- Clamp the needle between one fourth and one third of the distance from the suture end of the needle to the point of the needle. The needle should be recessed approximately 1/8 inch into the jaws of the needle holder.
- Pass the needle holder so that the point of the needle is toward the center of the surgeon's body.
- Place the free end of the suture over the back of the surgeon's hand. Place used needles on the needle counter or in another appropriate container (U.S. Army, 1988, pp. 104–105).

Applying and Removing a Pneumatic Tourniquet

General Guidelines

- Check the entire pneumatic tourniquet system for discrepancies, such as cracks or holes in the tubing, before each use.
- Ensure that the inner tube of the cuff is completely encased (AORN, 1992, *III*:13–1).
- Check the pressure source for adequate gas.
- Use an inert nonflammable gas such as nitrogen to inflate the cuff.
- Pressure in the tank should read at least 500 pounds/square inch.

Selecting the Tourniquet Cuff

- Assess the size of the patient's extremity and select a cuff that overlaps at the ends no more than 3 inches.

Applying the Tourniquet Cuff

- Unless contraindicated by the manufacturer's instructions, apply wrinkle-free padding before applying the tourniquet cuff.
- Position the cuff above the elbow or knee "at the point of maximum circumference of the limb" (AORN, 1992, *III*:13–2).
- Avoid an incomplete or overly aggressive seal of the cuff. An improper cuff seal may result in bruising, blistering, pinching, or necrosis of the skin.
- Secure the tourniquet by tying the cuff strings in a bow. Do not tie a knot. This interferes with removal, especially in an emergency situation.

- After applying the tourniquet cuff, do not rotate to a new position. Rotating the cuff after application leads to shearing forces, which may damage the underlying tissue (AORN, 1992, *III*:13–2).

Preparing and Draping the Extremity After Tourniquet Application

- Apply an impervious barrier around the cuff during the skin preparation.
- If preparation solutions seep under the cuff during the preparation, remove the cuff, dry the limb and the cuff, and then reapply the cuff.
- While draping the extremity, especially around the tourniquet cuff, do not puncture the cuff with the towel clip or other sharp object.

Preparing the Limb for Tourniquet Inflation

- If the surgeon wraps the limb before inflating the tourniquet cuff, depending on the size of the limb, use a 4- or 6-inch Esmarch or elastic (Ace) bandage.
- Starting with the hand or the foot, elevate and tightly wrap the limb toward the cuff.
- After wrapping, inflate the cuff.
- Unwrap the limb by reversing the procedure and rewind the bandage.
- Save the bandage for later use.

Inflating the Tourniquet

- Consider the patient's age and systolic blood pressure, the width of the tourniquet, and the circumference of the limb when selecting a tourniquet inflation pressure.
- As a guideline, in the healthy adult patient, 50 to 75 mm Hg above the systolic pressure for an arm and 100 to 150 mm Hg above the systolic pressure for a leg usually produce a bloodless field (AORN, 1992, *III*:13–2). Pressures are lower for children and for patients with impaired tissue perfusion.

Monitoring the Tourniquet Intraoperatively

- Ensure that the pressure gauge is clearly visible. Do not cover it with drapes.
- Check the cuff periodically during inflation for pressure fluctuations.
- Watch the tourniquet inflation time.
- As a general guideline, the tourniquet should stay inflated no longer than 1 hour for an arm and $1\frac{1}{2}$ hours for a leg in the healthy adult patient (AORN, 1992, *III*:13–2).

Removing the Tourniquet

- Do not deflate the tourniquet cuff until instructed by the surgeon.
- After the cuff is deflated, remove the cuff and padding, and inspect the skin for signs of chemical burn, bruising, blistering, pinching, and necrosis.

Documenting Tourniquet Use

- Location of the cuff
- Identification of the person who applied the cuff
- Cuff pressure and time of inflation and deflation
- Skin and tissue integrity under the cuff before and after the use of the pneumatic tourniquet
- Identification number of the specific tourniquet (AORN, 1992, III:13–3)

Applying and Removing the Electrosurgical Unit Dispersive Electrode

General Guidelines

- Before use, inspect the electrosurgical unit by testing the alarm system and looking for frayed wires and loose connections.
- Place the generator close enough to the sterile field to ensure that the active electrode cord is connected without tension.
- Use the electrosurgical unit at the lowest possible effective setting.
- Confirm orally with the operator the activation and settings.
- When higher than usual settings are requested, check for malfunction or loose connections. If no loose connections or malfunctions are found and high settings are still required, obtain another generator.
- Electrosurgical units are not usually used for patients with pacemakers owing to the potential for electrical interference with the pacemaker.
- To avoid possible fire, do not use electrosurgical units in the presence of flammable agents.
- Do not use extension cords on an electrosurgical unit generator (AORN, 1992, III:5–1—5–2).

Applying the Dispersive Electrode

- Ensure that the dispersive electrode has adequate gel for good conduction.
- Electrode size should provide adequate body contact and grounding.
- Place the grounding pad over a large muscle mass and as close to the wound site as possible.

- Do not apply the grounding pad over bony prominences, scar tissue, areas with large metal prosthetic implants (total hip replacements, internal rods, and plates), or excessively hairy areas.
- Shave hairy patients at the dispersive electrode site before applying the pad. This ensures good contact of the pad and gel with the skin.
- Apply the dispersive electrode with uniform contact with the skin.
- Do not place the dispersive electrode pad circumferentially on an extremity because of the potential for a tourniquet effect and decreased tissue perfusion.
- Protect the patient from a potential thermal injury by placing the grounding pad in areas where liquids do not accumulate.
- Do not place the grounding pad near electrocardiographic electrodes or rectal probes.
- Before and during the procedure, check to ensure that the patient is not touching metal objects such as intravenous poles and stirrup holders.
- If contact with metal objects unavoidably occurs, insulate the object with a nonconductive material such as foam, rubber, or cloth.
- During the procedure, check the grounding pad for tenting and puckering, and reposition as necessary (AORN, 1992, *III*:5–2).

Removing the Dispersive Electrode

- Do not remove the electrode until the dressing has been applied and the drapes taken off the patient.
- Carefully and slowly peel the dispersive electrode from the patient's skin.
- Assess the application site for signs of electrical burns.
- Check the patient for burns caused by an alternative exit pathway of electrical current, particularly at the application sites for electrocardiographic leads.

Monitoring the Active Electrode

- The scrub person monitors the active electrode during surgery.
- Before use, inspect the active electrode for damage, especially if it is reusable. Look for frayed wires and check that the tip fits tightly in the pencil.
- Hand the active electrode cord from the sterile field without loops and twists.
- During the procedure, remove charred tissue from the blades and tips of the active electrode.
- When the active electrode is not in use, place it in a clean, dry, nonconductive, and highly visible area during procedures.
- Do not allow the active electrode to contact metal clamps or to lie on exposed patient skin (AORN, 1992, *III*:5–2).

Documenting Electrosurgery

- Patient's preoperative and postoperative skin condition at the dispersive electrode site
- Area of placement of the dispersive electrode
- Identification of the electrosurgical unit and its settings (AORN, 1992, *III*:4–1)

Preparing Electrical Instruments and Equipment for Use

- Prepare and operate electrical instruments and equipment according to the manufacturer's instructions.
- Inspect electrical instruments and equipment before use.
- Connect attachments to the electrical instrument and test the unit before use.
- Avoid accidental activation of the unit by ensuring that triggers are in the safety position and on-off switches are in the off position when changing attachments and plugging in the instrument (AORN, 1992, *III*:9–5).
- Check outlets and switch plates for damage.
- Examine cords and plugs for fraying or other damage. Damaged outlets and switch plates, as well as frayed cords and plugs, may result in excessive current leakage and cause patient or personnel injury (AORN, 1992, *III*:7–4).
- Eliminate the potential for tripping or accidental unplugging of the equipment by laying cords flat on the floor (AORN, 1992, *III*:7–4).
- Watch for pooled fluids on the floor.

Preparing Air-Powered Instruments for Use

- Inspect and test air-powered instruments before use.
- Ensure that the manufacturer's instructions are followed when an air-powered instrument is used.
- Meticulously inspect hoses before using the air-powered instrument (AORN, 1992, *III*:9–5).
- Prevent injury to patient and personnel by connecting attachments and testing the unit before use.
- Avoid accidental activation when changing attachments by placing the triggering mechanism in the safety position (AORN, 1992, *III*:9–5).
- Use medical-grade compressed air or compressed dry nitrogen (99.97% pure) for air-powered instruments.
- Check the tank before use. At least 1000 pounds/square inch should register on the tank pressure gauge.
- Do not set pounds per square inch unless the instrument is running.
- Use the manufacturer's recommended pounds per square inch when using an air-powered instrument.

- Do not automatically exceed the recommended pounds per square inch if the instrument operation is sluggish or erratic.

Preparing the Hyperthermia or Hypothermia Unit for Use

- Before using the hypothermia or hyperthermia unit, ensure that the fluid reservoir is filled according to the manufacturer's instructions.
- Check controls to ensure proper functioning. Lights should illuminate when the unit is on.
- Inspect the blanket surfaces and tubing for holes and kinks before placing the blanket on the OR bed.
- Attach the blanket tubing to the hypothermia or hyperthermia unit.
- Set the controls to the desired heating or cooling temperature and activate the unit.
- As the unit pumps fluid through the tubing and blanket, check for leaks.
- After checking the blanket and tubing for leaks, place the blanket on the OR bed.
- Unless the blanket is designed for direct skin contact, cover the blanket with an absorbable pad or sheet.
- Prevent folds and creases in the blanket that may hinder the proper flow of fluid through the blanket and cause hot or cold spots on the blanket's surface (AORN, 1992, *III:7*–3).
- During use of the unit, periodically assess unit functioning.
- Feel for excessive heat or cold radiating from the tubing and the blanket.
- Check the temperature controls to ensure that they are set for the correct temperature.

Applying Dressings
Preparing the Incision

- Before removing drapes, the scrub person cleans the incision site with a wet sterile sponge or towel to remove dried preparation solution, blood, other body fluid, and tissue.
- Dry the skin around the incision after cleaning.

Applying the Dressing

- Avoid using radiopaque sponges for dressings.
- Hold the dressing in place with one hand and remove the drapes from the incision site with the other hand.

Applying the Tape

- The circulating nurse applies the tape.
- If the surgeon applies the tape, he or she should remove the gloves to prevent cross-contamination.

- Secure the dressing in place with tape.
- Do not stretch the skin while applying the tape.

Assisting With the Application of Casts and Splints
Preparing the Operating Room

- Protect the OR by spreading a disposable plastic or fabric sheet on the floor around the OR bed.
- Protect the OR bed by covering exposed areas with a suitable draping material.

Preparing the Casting Materials and Equipment

- Select the plaster rolls, cut the padding, and obtain other materials, such as stockinet and Webril, according to the physician's preference (Table 4).
- Place a plastic liner bag in the plaster bucket and fill with lukewarm water, about 70°F to 80°F (U.S. Army, 1967, p. 94).

Padding the Cast

- For a close-fitting and well-contoured cast, use the stockinet for padding material.
- Do not use it alone if the patient has an acute fracture or excessive swelling or immediately after an operation.
- If the stockinet is used without padding, document this fact on the cast with an indelible ink pen.
- The surgeon may elect to wrap sheet cotton or Webril bandage over the stockinet. If Webril is used, wrap it smoothly in one to three layers with the turns overlapping about one half the width of the bandage.
- Pad bony prominences to reduce the risk of skin breakdown after the cast has been applied.
- If necessary, place heavy felt pieces over bony prominences (U.S. Army, 1967, p. 94).

Preparing the Plaster Bandage Roll

- When dipping the plaster roll, hold it in a vertical position. This allows air to escape through the core of the roll.
- Dip the roll in the lukewarm water for approximately 5 seconds or until the water stops bubbling.
- Hold the roll at each end and squeeze. Do not wring the water out of the roll. Squeeze at the ends while pushing toward the center.
- Leave enough water in the roll to delay drying, thus ensuring proper application before the plaster sets.
- Pass the plaster roll to the surgeon (U.S. Army, 1967, p. 94).

TABLE 4
Basic Cast Supplies and Equipment

Name	Description
Cotton bandages, plaster of Paris impregnated	Available in widths of 2, 3, 4, and 6 inches; used as the basic material to form casts
Splints, plaster of Paris impregnated for leg and arm	Length and width are short and narrow (3 × 15 inches), short and wide (4 × 15 inches), and long and wide (5 × 30 inches); used to reinforce casts and reduce the time for application
Stockinet	Tubular, seamless ribbed knit material of natural color; available in widths of 3, 6, 10, and 12 inches; thin padding next to cast; helps to make close-fitting, contoured cast
Cotton wadding	Available in widths of 5 inches × 6 yards; padding for casts
Webril bandage	Available in 2, 3, 4, and 6 inches × 4 yards; used as padding
Felt bandages	Available in large white rolls and can be split into the thickness and cut into the size and shape required; used for padding bony prominences
Electrical cutter	Available with 2- and 2½-inch blades; used for cutting casts; may have vacuum attached to confine plaster dust
Cast knives	Various sizes available; the compound dental knife with detachable No. 21 blade is commonly used
Spreaders, benders, scissors, and pliers	Spreaders used to spread the edges of casts; benders, for bending back the adges; bandage scissors, for cutting materials; ordinary pliers, for tightening blades on cast cutter
Plaster cart	Used for containing supplies and preparing casts
Metal splints, padded	Used for splinting finger fractures
Bucket, 8 quart	Used for dipping plaster products
Pillows, plastic covered	Used for elevating limbs after casting

Adapted from U.S. Army. (1967). *Orthopedic specialist: TM 8–231, AFM 160–6* (pp. 93–97). U.S. Departments of the Army and the Air Force. Baltimore: U.S. Army Publications Center.

Preparing the Plaster Splint

- Select the number and size of splint sheets according to the surgeon's preference, dip in the water, and rapidly withdraw them.
- Place the splints on a work table and smooth out with the palm of the hand.
- Draw each side of the splint through the index and middle fingers and pass to the surgeon.

- Give the surgeon a plaster bandage to tie the splint (U.S. Army, 1967, p. 94).

Molding the Cast

- The surgeon will rub and mold the cast over the contour of the body part. During this process, he or she may apply a few drops of water to make the surface smooth.
- If plaster crumbs develop, remove the crumbs with water; this prevents the formation of rough spots in the cast.
- Molding continues until the plaster begins to set, or until the plaster is no longer glossy or creamy.
- Ventilate the cast to dissipate heat.
- Do not cover the cast (U.S. Army, 1967, p. 94).

Finishing the Cast

- The surgeon finishes the cast by trimming it with a cast knife.
- After trimming the cast, fold the stockinet over the edges of the cast.
- A plaster splint is applied over the folded edge, and the splint is smoothed over.
- Place the patient's casted extremity on a pillow.
- To prevent cast denting, protect the cast from contacting rough surfaces (U.S. Army, 1967, p. 96).

Removing the Cast

- Most casts are removed with an electrical cast cutter.
- Remove the cast outside the restricted areas of the surgical suite to confine plaster dust.
- Use a cast cutter with an attached vacuum to confine plaster dust that is generated during the removal process.
- When removing the cast, exercise care in cutting over bony prominences or areas where the bones are close to the surface of the skin, such as the shin.
- Look for notes on the cast that indicate areas of light padding (U.S. Army, 1967, pp. 96–97).
- If an electrical cast cutter is not available, remove the cast by soaking it in water until it becomes soft.
- After the cast is softened, unravel it, starting with the end of the last roll applied.

Precautions

- Do not place circular dressing of cloth, adhesive, moleskin, elastic bandage, or any material other than acceptable padding under the cast.
- Use the palm of the hand, not the fingertips, to hold a wet cast.
- Because plaster generates heat while setting, expose the cast to air while it is drying (U.S. Army, 1967, p. 97).

Discharge Instructions for the Patient

CAST CARE (U.S. Army, 1967, p. 97)
- Do not walk on new walking casts for 24 hours.
- Keep all casts dry.
- Do not alter casts.
- Do not remove casts.
- Do not put foreign objects inside casts.

PREVENTION OF COMPLICATIONS
- To prevent swelling when a cast is applied to a limb, elevate the limb for 2 days.
- Report pressure points.
- If a cast becomes soft or broken, return for repairs.
- If a cast becomes too loose, return for a new one.
- If in doubt, return to have the cast checked.
- Follow the physician's orders.

ADMINISTERING DRUGS AND SOLUTIONS

The perioperative nurse demonstrates competency to administer drugs and solutions by
- Visiting the patient and the family before surgery to obtain a medication history
- Verifying patient identification, the correct drug or solution, the correct dosage, the correct route, and the correct time for administration
- Knowing potential drug reactions, complications, and contraindications
- Having available specific antidotes and other emergency drugs and equipment
- Gathering prescribed medications and necessary supplies and equipment
- Using resources as needed (e.g., *AMA Drug Evaluations* [American Medical Association, 1984], FDA Drug Bulletin, *Physicians' Desk Reference* [1992], hospital formulary, manufacturer's product information, and other selected pharmacology texts and journal articles)
- Communicating with the hospital pharmacist as needed
- Preparing and administering drugs and solutions according to institutional policy, manufacturer's recommendations, and federal and state regulations
- Verifying the drug, the doses, and the route of administration with the physician and the scrub person before transferring a drug to the sterile field
- Performing procedures for charging the patient for drugs and solutions administered

- Obtaining the patient's consent for the use of experimental drugs
- Disposing of needles, syringes, glassware, and contaminated material according to accepted guidelines
- Verifying verbal orders before administration
- Questioning orders that appear to be erroneous
- Documenting the drug or solution, its dosage, the time and route of administration, and the name of the individual who prepared and administered the substance

Taking the Preoperative Medication History
Health Perception–Health Management Pattern
- What medications are you presently taking?
- What do these medications do for you?
- Do they seem to work?
- What medications have you taken in the past?
- Did they seem to work for you?
- Do you have any allergies to drugs, foods, chemicals, or other materials such as tape or iodine?
- Do you use alcohol, tobacco, or recreational drugs?
- On a scale of 1 to 10, rate your compliance with (how well you stick to) your medication regimen (10 being 100% compliance).

Nutritional-Metabolic Pattern
- Age
- Weight pounds _____ kilograms _____
- Height
- Abnormal laboratory values or test results
- Do you take any special foods with, before, or after your medications?
- Do you have any problems associated with your medications? Skin problems? Dental or gum problems? Difficulty healing?

Elimination Pattern
- Have your medications caused any problems with elimination (constipation, polyuria, diarrhea)?
- Do you use over-the-counter laxatives?

Activity-Exercise Pattern
- Have you had a change in energy related to your medications?
- Are you able to take your medications, or do you need assistance?
- Functional level related to the ability to self-medicate:
  Level I: Requires use of equipment or devices
  Level II: Requires assistance or supervision from another person

Level III: Requires assistance or supervision from another person and equipment or devices

Level IV: Is dependent and does not participate

Sleep-Rest Pattern

- Have your medications changed your sleep habits?
- Do you have any nightmares or dreams associated with your medications?
- Do you use any aids to sleep (alcohol, medications, foods)?

Cognitive-Perceptual Pattern

- Have you experienced any changes related to your medications? Changes in vision, hearing, memory, decision making, and associated pain or discomfort?

Self-perception–Self-concept Pattern

- Have you noticed any changes in how you feel about yourself since you have been taking medications?
- Have you had any changes in your body, such as weight gain or loss, enlarged breasts, and fluid retention?
- Have you had a change in your attitude, such as anger, depression, and fear?

Role-Relationship Pattern

- If need be, is there someone at home who can help you with your medications?
- Has taking medications interfered with your ability to perform your life roles (wife/husband, parent, jobholder, and so on)?

Sexuality-Reproductive Pattern

- Has your medication altered your sexual drive or changed your sexual relationship?
- If appropriate: Do you use contraception? When was your last menstrual period? Are there any menstrual problems related to medications?

Coping–Stress Tolerance Pattern

- Do you use any medications, herbs, folk remedies, or alcohol to help you cope with stress?
- Are these methods effective?
- Do you presently use or have a history of using recreational drugs?

Values-Beliefs Pattern

- Does taking your medication interfere with your religious beliefs or values? If so, how? Is there interference with your cultural or ethnic beliefs or values? If so, how?

Perioperative Medications

Key Terms (Tables 5 to 11)
Examples (Tables 12 to 15)
Medications That Interact With Heparin (Table 16)

Supplies and Equipment for Medication Administration

Syringes

- Use syringes with needles to reconstitute powders with a diluent and for aspirating a solution or suspension from a vial or an ampule. Syringe selection (size and type) is dependent on the medication being prepared and dispensed.
- Because the amount of medication varies according to its type and function, use judgment in selecting syringe size. Generally, a 10 ml syringe is used for injection of local anesthetics and for reconstituting powders with diluent. Larger syringes are usually

TABLE 5
Key Terms for Anti-infective Drugs

Antibiotic	A chemical compound produced by microorganisms, which can inhibit the growth of, or kill, other organisms
Bactericidal	A compound having direct action on bacteria that results in their destruction or death
Bacteriostatic	A compound that inhibits the growth or multiplication of bacteria
Gram stain	A method of staining bacteria that is used to identify various types of bacteria
Gram-negative	A characteristic of certain microorganisms whereby they lose their initial stain when treated with a decolorizing solution used in the Gram stain procedure
Gram-positive	A characteristic whereby certain microorganisms stained with crystal violet and iodine and retain they stain after decolorizing
Active immunity	Immunity that is attained by prior exposure to a pathogen or to its antigen, which stimulated production of specific antibodies; also known as acquired immunity
Passive immunity	Protection against a pathogen and its toxins by transfer of antibodies produced in the body of another person or animal that has been actively immunized
Acquired resistance	A state in which an organism that was once sensitive to an anti-infective drug has developed the ability to remain unaffected by that drug
Congenital resistance	An inborn ability to remain unaffected by certain anti-infective drugs
Microbial resistance	The ability of a microorganism to withstand the effects of anti-infective drugs

TABLE 6
Key Terms for Anticoagulant Therapy

Ecchymosis	A small spot caused by bleeding in the skin or mucous membranes, forming a round or irregular purple patch
Embolus	A clot carried by the blood from a larger vessel to a smaller vessel, which becomes blocked
Hematoma	A localized collection of blood in a space, organ, or tissue
Petechia	A tiny red spot caused by the escape of a small amount of blood
Phlebothrombosis	The presence of blood clots in a vein without inflammation
Thrombophlebitis	Inflammation and clotting within a vein
Thrombus	A solid mass of clotted blood in a vessel or in the heart

TABLE 7
Key Terms for Local Anesthetics

Topical analgesia	Application of a cream, ointment, or fluid for the purpose of anesthetizing the skin or mucous membrane
Infiltration anesthesia	Injection of solutions of local anesthesia into tissue to bring the anesthetic into contact with nerve endings in the intracutaneous, subcutaneous, and deeper structures and keep these sensitive nerve terminals from transmitting pain impulses
Field block	A form of infiltration anesthesia in which the sensory nerve pathways from the operative field are blocked off by a circular ring of subcutaneously injected solution
Central nerve block	Block that affects the roots of nerves at various points close to their origin in the spinal cord
Peripheral nerve block	Block affecting the trunks of specific nerves such as the sciatic-femoral, ulnar, or intercostal nerves, or the brachial plexus
Intravenous regional block	Local anesthesia of an arm or a leg by injection of local anesthetic into a vein after exsanguination and application of a pneumatic tourniquet

more difficult to control than smaller ones because greater force is needed for aspiration and injection.

- When preparing small doses of potentially dangerous medications, such as heparin or epinephrine, it is best to use a 1 ml insulin or tuberculin syringe to ensure accurate dosage.

TABLE **8**
Key Terms Associated With the Administration of Ophthalmic Agents

Aphakia	Absence of the lens of the eye; may be congenital or occur after injury or surgery.
Adrenergic agents	Medications that constrict the vessels of the eye, thereby reducing the rate at which aqueous fluid is formed within the eye. In addition, the outflow of fluid may be increased. This mechanism, which is not clearly understood, helps to lower the intraocular pressure.
Cholinergic agents	Medications that directly or indirectly cause the sphincter muscles of the iris and of the ciliary body to contract.
Cycloplegic agent	Medication that causes paralysis of accomodation by relaxing the ciliary muscles of the eye.
Gonioscopy	Examination of the filtration angle of the anterior eye chamber with an optical instrument designed to visualize the area and determine anterior chamber width.
Hyperosmotic agents	Medications that increase the osmotic pressure of the blood plasma to a point above that of the aqueous humor and the vitreous body of the eye. Intraocular fluid then follows the osmotic gradient into the hyperosmotic plasma. The loss of fluid leads to a reduction in intraocular pressure.
Inner canthus	The angle at the nasal end of the opening between the eyelids.
Miotic agent	Medication that causes constriction of the pupil.
Mydriatic agent	Medication that causes dilatation of the pupil of the eye.
Tonometry	The process of using a tonometer to measure intraocular pressure.
Trabecula	Supporting fibers of connecting tissue.

TYPES OF SYRINGES
- Luer-Lok tip. This syringe has a tip that locks over the needle hub. It is used whenever pressure is exerted to inject or aspirate fluid. Sizes range from 2 to 60 ml.
- Luer-slip tip. This syringe has a plain tip that may not provide a secure connection on a needle hub. It is not recommended for preparing medications but may be needed for administering medications through catheters and ports. Sizes range from 1 to 60 ml.
- Ring control. This syringe has a Luer-Lok tip with a finger hold and thumb hold. It is ideal for injection of local anesthetics. The syringe allows firm control when injecting with only one hand. Sizes range from 3 to 10 ml.

TABLE 9

Key Terms Associated With the Administration of Otic Medications

Auricle or pinna	External part of the ear composed of cartilage and covered by skin.
Cochlea	Winding cone-shaped tube forming a portion of the inner ear.
Eustachian tube	Tube that brings air to the middle ear, thus equalizing pressure on both sides of the tympanic membrane.
External auditory canal	Includes the outer portion of the ear, the canal, and the tympanic membrane.
Inner ear or labyrinth	A system of tubes and spaces within a hollowed-out temporal bone, collectively called the bony labyrinth.
Mastoid air cells	Air-filled spaces in the temporal bone. The middle ear communicates posteriorly with the mastoid ear cells.
Ossicles	Three bones of the ear: malleolus, incus, and stapes.
Tragus	Cartilaginous projection in front of the exterior meatus of the ear.
Tympanic membrane	The eardrum, which divides the meatus and the middle ear cavity.

TABLE 10

Key Terms for Skin Medications

Antihistamine	Antagonizes the effects of free histamine on the skin and its blood vessels and thus relieves the cutaneous signs and symptoms of allergy
Anti-infective	Used to treat or prevent skin or mucous membrane infection by pathogenic microbes (e.g., antimicrobials, antifungals, antiseptics, antibacterials)
Anti-inflammatory	Used to reduce skin inflammation and relieve its signs and symptoms
Antiseptic	Chemical substance that kills microorganisms and prevents their growth
Demulcent	Used to coat the skin and mucous membranes, thereby providing mechanical protection against irritation of these surfaces
Depilatory	Chemical used to remove hair
Detergent	Used to clean the skin; usually has some antiseptic properties
Dusting powder	Inert substance applied to the skin to protect the irritated surface or to absorb excessive moisture
Emollient	Oily or fatty substance used to prevent the evaporation of water and drying of the skin
Proteolytic enzymes	Chemical substance applied to the skin to speed the breakdown of necrotic tissue in ulcerated or burned skin areas (e.g., for chemical débridement of dead tissue)

TABLE **11**
Key Terms for Contrast Media

Arteriogram	Radiographic study of an artery to determine arterial perfusion, size, and shape.
Arthrogram	Radiographic study of a joint cavity to outline the contour of the joint.
Cholangiogram	Radiographic study of the bile ducts.
Cystogram	Radiographic study of the bladder.
Cystourethrogram	Radiographic study of the bladder and ureters.
Diskogram	Radiographic study of intervertebral disks.
Hysterosalpingogram	Study of the uterus and fallopian tubes after injection of radiopaque material into those structures.
Pyelogram	Radiographic study of the ureter and renal pelvis. For an IV pyelogram, the contrast medium is given intravenously and an x-ray film of the urinary tract is taken while the material is excreted. This provides important information about the structure and function of the kidney, ureter, and bladder.

SYRINGES FOR IRRIGATION
- Bulb syringe with barrel. This syringe has a rubber or plastic bulb attached to the neck of the barrel. It is used for irrigation in many types of procedure. Sizes have a solution capacity ranging from $\frac{1}{4}$ to 4 ounces.
- Bulb syringe without barrel. This syringe is also known as the ear syringe. It is a one-piece bulb that tapers to a blunt end. It is used for irrigating the ear, the eye, or other small structures.

Needles

The size of a needle is designated by length and gauge. Gauge is the outside diameter of the needle. The bevel of a needle is its sloped edge. Commonly used sizes include
- $\frac{1}{2}$ inch × 30 gauge for local anesthesia in plastic surgery
- $\frac{3}{4}$ inch × 25 gauge for local anesthesia or conjunctival injection
- $1\frac{1}{2}$ inches × 22 gauge for subcutaneous or intramuscular injection
- 2 inches × 16 or 18 gauge for preparation of medications and solutions
- 4 inches × 20 or 22 gauge; spinal needles used for deep injection of local anesthetic

Diluent
- 0.9% sodium chloride. This preparation is designed for parenteral use only after the addition of drugs that require dilution

TABLE 12

Common Preoperative Medications

Drug	Usual Preoperative Dose*
Sedatives and Hypnotics	
Pentobarbital sodium (Nembutal)	50–200 mg PO
Secobarbital sodium (Seconal)	200–300 mg PO
Chloral hydrate	0.5–1 g PO
Tranquilizers	
Chlorpromazine hydrochloride (Thorazine)	20–50 mg PO, 12.5–25 mg IM
Hydroxyzine hydrochloride (Vistaril)	50–100 mg PO, 25–100 mg IM
Diazepam (Valium)	5–10 mg PO or IM
Promethazine hydrochloride (Phenergan)	50 mg PO, 25–50 mg IM
Narcotics (Opiates)	
Meperidine hydrochloride (Demerol)	50–100 mg IM or SC
Morphine sulfate	5–15 mg IM or SC
Hydromorphone hydrochloride (Dilaudid)	2–4 mg PO or IM
Anticholinergics	
Atropine sulfate	0.4–0.6 mg PO, SC, IM, or IV
Glycopyrrolate (Robinul)	0.002 mg/pound (0.004 mg/kg) of body weight IM
Scopolamine (hyoscine)	0.3–0.6 mg IM or SC

*PO, orally; IM, intramuscularly; SC, subcutaneously; IV, intravenously.
From Ignatavius, D., Bayne, M. V. (1991). *Medical-surgical nursing: A nursing process approach* (p. 451). Philadelphia: W. B. Saunders.

or that must be dissolved in an aqueous vehicle before injection. Do not use unless the solution is clear and the container is undamaged. When diluting or dissolving drugs, mix thoroughly and use promptly.

- Bacteriostatic water for injection. Used as a diluting or dissolving agent according to the drug manufacturer's recommendation.

Preparing Medications and Solutions From Ampules and Vials

Task Standard

The perioperative nurse prepares medications and solutions from ampules and vials in a manner that

- Prevents contamination of the ampule or vial contents
- Maintains sterility of the needle and syringe parts
- Ensures accurate dosage of medication or solution

Precautions

Monitor respiratory status.
Monitor level of anxiety; encourage verbalization and relaxation.

Maintain NPO status and assess for gastrointestinal upset or nausea.

Promote relaxation by dimming lights and instructing the patient on the importance of relaxation.

Give deep intramuscular injection with 1- or 1½-inch needle.

Monitor blood pressure and respiratory status.

Monitor blood pressure and heart rate.
Monitor hydration and maintain NPO status.

Supplies and Equipment
- Appropriate-sized syringe and needle
- Protective pad for opening ampule
- Sharps container
- Diluent
- 0.9% sodium chloride injection
- Bacteriostatic water for injection

Removing Medication or Solution From an Ampule
- Identify the type, dose, and expiration date of the medication.
- Tap the ampule lightly and quickly until the fluid leaves the neck of the ampule and flows to the lower chamber.
- Place a gauze or alcohol pad around the neck of the ampule. This helps protect the fingers when the ampule is broken. Do not remove the alcohol pad from its wrapper. Alcohol may leak into the ampule.

TABLE **13**
Frequently Used Local Anesthetics

Generic Name	Trade Name
Benzocaine	Americaine, Anesthesin
Mepivacaine hydrochloride	Carbocaine
Prilocaine hydrochloride	Citanest hydrochloride
Cocaine hydrochloride topical solution	—
Bupivacaine hydrochloride	Marcaine hydrochloride, Sensorcaine
Chloroprocaine hydrochloride	Nesacaine, Nesacaine CE
Procaine hydrochloride	Novocain
Tetracaine	Pontocaine hydrochloride, Anacel
Lidocaine	Xylocaine

*Epinephrine-containing solutions have a duration of 1½ to 2 times as long as plain solutions.

- Snap the neck of the ampule along the prescored line. Direct the snapping motion away from the body. While snapping the top off, avoid shattering the glass. If it is suspected that glass has entered the ampule, discard it and start again.
- Hold the ampule upside down or place it on a flat surface. The ampule may be held upside down without danger of spillage as long as the needle tip or shaft does not touch the ampule. After the needle touches the ampule, surface tension breaks down and fluid leaks out.
- Insert the needle into the ampule without touching the rim.
- Keep the needle tip below the surface of the liquid and quickly draw up the medication without injecting air into the ampule. Injection of air forces the fluid out of the ampule. Because the fluid in the ampule is immediately displaced by air, there is no resistance to its withdrawal.
- Confirm the type, dose, and expiration date of the medication with the scrub person.
- Dispense the medication onto the sterile field. The scrub person should position the medication receptacle at the edge of the field or hold it so that the solution can be released without contamination.

Duration of Action*	Precautions
—	Topical; used on broken and mucous membrane
60–120 min	Infiltration and conduction; plain, 300 mg; with epinephrine, 500 mg
30–120 min	Infiltration and conduction; plain, 600 mg; with epinephrine, 600 mg
—	Topical, 200 mg
120–240 min	Infiltration and conduction; plain, 175 mg; with epinephrine, 225 mg
15–30 min	Infiltration and conduction; plain, 800 mg; with epinephrine, 1000 mg
15–30 min	Infiltration and conduction; plain, 1000 mg; with epinephrine, 600 mg
120–240 min	Infiltration and conduction; plain, 100 mg; with epinephrine, 200 mg
30–120 min	Infiltration and conduction; plain, 300 mg; with epinephrine, 500 mg

- Dispose of the needle, syringe, and gauze or alcohol pad. This protects other personnel from inadvertent injury from the needle or glass slivers. Discard unused medication.

Removing Medication or Solution From a Vial
- Identify the type, dose, and expiration date of the medication.
- Remove the plastic or metal cap covering the top of the unused vial. If the vial is a multiple-dose vial and has been used previously, wipe the rubber seal with alcohol before and after each use. This removes surface bacteria, dust, and dried solution from the stopper.
- Prepare the syringe with as much air as solution to be removed from the vial. As medication is removed, replacement with air is required to prevent a buildup of negative pressure.
- Insert the needle, with the bevel pointing up, through the center of the vial. The center of the vial is thinner and is designed for penetration. Keep the bevel up to prevent cutting a rubber core from the seal.
- Inject air into the vial. While injecting air, hold onto the plunger. The plunger may be forced backward by air pressure within the vial. For vials with dry medication, diluent is used to replace air, thereby creating positive pressure in the vial.

TABLE 14

Common Intraoperative Anti-infectives

Generic Name	Trade Name	Adult Dosage
Polymyxin B sulfate	Aerosporin	1.5–2.5 mg/kg in divided doses
Amikacin sulfate	Amikin	IV; 15–30 mg/kg/d q8–12h
Ampicillin	—	IV; 150–200 mg/kg/d in divided doses
Cefazolin sodium	Ancef, Kefzol	2 g q4h
Azlocillin	Azlin	IV; 3 g q4h
Bacitracin	—	Irrigation; 50,000 U in 1000 ml of 0.9% sodium chloride
Cefoperazone sodium	Cefobid	IV; 2 g q12h
Cefotetan disodium	Cefotan	IV; 1–3 g q12h
Clindamycin	Cleocin hydrochloride	IV; 150–900 mg q8h
Chloramphenicol	Chloromycetin	IV; 50 mg/kg/d
Erythromycin glucceptate	Ilotycin glucceptate	IV; 250–500 mg q4–6h
Gentamicin	Garamycin	IV; 3–5 mg/kg/d in divided doses
Cefamandole nafate	Mandol	IV; 0.5–2 g q4h
Cefoxitin sodium	Mefoxin	IV; 2 g q4h
Mezlocillin sodium	Mezlin	IV; 3 mg q4h
Penicillin G	—	IV; usually greater than 20,000,000 U/d
Methicillin sodium	Staphcillin	IV; 1–2 g q4h
Ticarcillin disodium	Ticar	IV; 3 g q4h
Vancomycin	Vancocin	IV; 1 g q12h
Cerfuroxime	Zinacef	IV; 1.5 g q8h

TABLE 15

Frequently Used Anticholinergic Agents

Cycloplegic Agent	Recommended Doses
Atropine sulfate	1 to 2 drops of a 1% solution
Cyclopentolate hydrochloride	2 drops of 0.5% solution or 1 drop of a 1% solution
Homatropine	1 to 2 drops of a 1 to 2% solution
Tropicamide	1 to 2 drops of a 0.5 to 1% solution

TABLE **16**
Medications That Interact With Heparin*

Agent	Potential Effect
Anticoagulants, oral	Prolonged prothrombin time
Antihistamines	Partial antagonist of anticoagulant action of heparin
Aspirin and other salicylates	Inhibition of platelet adhesiveness and aggregation
Contraceptives, oral	Estrogen-containing contraceptives may reduce the concentration of antithrombin III and result in increased thrombotic activity
Digitalis glycosides	Partial antagonistic action of heparin
Dextran	Inhibition of platelet adhesiveness
Dipyridamole (Persantine)	
Indomethacin (Indocin)	
Ibuprofen (Motrin)	
Streptokinase	May partially antagonize anticoagulant action of heparin
Tetracyclines	
Urokinase	

*Heparin sodium is a common drug used in vascular and cardiac procedures and in selected cases involving injury or infection of limbs and pelvic organs. Frequently, patients requiring such surgical intervention are taking a variety of medications for one or more coexisting conditions or diseases (e.g., cardiac disease, arthritis, asthma, hay fever). Untoward effects can occur when heparin is administered in conjunction with other medications.
Adapted from Govoni, L. E., Hayes, J. E. (1985). *Drugs and nursing implications* (p. 628). East Norwalk, Conn: Appleton-Century-Crofts.

- Invert the vial with the nondominant hand while grasping the syringe barrel and plunger with the thumb and forefinger of the dominant hand. Inverting the vial allows fluid to settle in the lower section of the vial.
- Allow air pressure to fill the syringe; pull back slightly on the plunger if necessary. Positive pressure in the vial causes the syringe to fill.
- After the correct volume is obtained, withdraw the needle from the vial.
- For multiple-dose vials, prepare a label that includes the date and time of mixing and the concentration per milliliter.
- Confirm the type, dose, and expiration date of the medication with the scrub person.
- Dispense the medication onto the sterile field. The scrub person should position the medication receptacle at the edge of the field or hold it so that the solution can be released without contamination.
- Dispose of the needle and syringe in an appropriate container.

Applying Skin Medications

Task Standard

The perioperative nurse applies topical medications to ensure proper penetration and absorption.

Purpose of Skin Medications

- Prevention or treatment of inflammation, discomfort, or infection
- Protection of the suture line or other skin surface
- Provision of local anesthesia over the skin surface

Supplies and Equipment

- Desired cream, ointment, or solution
- Sterile gloves
- Tongue blade or cotton-tipped applicators
- Dry sterile dressing
- Tape (paper or plastic)

Assessing the Patient

- Inspect the site of application for lesions, reddened areas, signs of infection, and breaks in skin or membranes.

Applying the Topical Ointment or Cream

- Don sterile gloves.
- Wash the application site to remove microorganisms, blood, debris, and fluids.
- Dry the application site. Moisture can interfere with application of the medication and hinder absorption of the medication.
- Apply the medication.
  1. Place the desired amount of medication on the sterile gauze.
  2. Apply the medication with a sterile tongue blade onto the suture line or desired skin surface. If a gloved finger is used for application, a fresh sterile glove should be donned. Glove powder should be removed.
  3. Avoid rubbing the skin, which may cause irritation, disruption of the suture line, or bleeding.
- Apply a dry sterile gauze or dressing as desired and secure with paper or plastic tape.

Applying an Aerosol Spray

- Shake the can vigorously, which mixes the contents and propellant to ensure a fine and even spray.
- Protect the patient's eyes and face from the spray by having the patient turn his or her head or by covering the face with a towel.
- Hold the can the recommended distance from the skin, usually 6 to 12 inches.

- Spray the desired area and allow it to dry before applying dressing or tape. This prevents the product from being removed by the dressing or tape.
- Cover the area with dressing as desired by the physician. Covering may help maintain the application on the skin.

Precautions
- Apply the least amount of medication that will obtain the desired effect. Excessive application of creams, ointments, or powders can result in skin irritation.

Administering Ophthalmic Medications
Task Standard
The perioperative nurse administers ocular solutions and ointments in a manner that
- Prevents injury to the eye
- Maintains the sterility of droppers, tubes, or medication containers

Purpose of Ophthalmic Applications
- Dilatation of the pupil for remeasurement of lens refraction or visualization of internal eye structures
- Paralysis of lens muscles for measurement of lens refraction
- Prevention or relief of local irritation or infection of the eye
- Local treatment of an increase in intraocular pressure
- Maintenance of lubrication of the cornea or the conjunctiva

Supplies and Equipment
- Desired ointment, eyedrop, or insert
- Gloves to protect the hands from purulent drainage or blood
- Cotton ball, gauze, or tissue
- Eye pad and tape for dressing if needed

Assessing the Patient
- Inspect the site of application for drainage, reddened areas, and encrusted areas.

Preparing the Patient
- Position the patient in a supine or a semi-Fowler position. These positions provide access to the eye and minimize drainage of medication through the lacrimal duct.
- If the eyelids are covered with crust or drainage, clean with sterile water or saline solution. Soak crust with warm solution if it is dry and difficult to remove. Soaking allows easy removal of crust and drainage that may harbor microorganisms. Always wipe

from the inner to the outer canthus. This prevents carrying debris to the lacrimal duct.
- Place the thumb and index finger near the margin of the lower eyelid immediately below the eyelashes, and exert downward pressure over the bony prominence of the cheek. Ask the patient to look upward while this is being done. This maneuver provides exposure of the lower conjunctival sac while retraction against the bony orbit prevents pressure and trauma to the eyeball. Upward eye motion retracts the cornea up and away from the conjunctival sac and reduces stimulation of the blink reflex.

Instilling Eyedrops

- Hold the dropper in the dominant hand about 1 to 2 cm above the conjunctival sac. This prevents dropper contact with the eyeball.
- Instill the prescribed number of drops into the eye. If the patient blinks and drops do not enter the eye, repeat the procedure. The conjunctival sac normally holds 1 to 2 drops.
- When administering drops that cause a systemic effect, protect the fingers with gloves or a tissue and apply gentle pressure to the patient's nasolacrimal duct for 30 to 60 seconds. This prevents absorption of the medication into the systemic circulation and prevents overflow of the drops into the nasopharyngeal passage.

Instilling Eye Ointment

- Have the patient look down to reduce the blinking reflex during ointment instillation.
- Hold the applicator above the lid margin and apply a thin stream of ointment evenly along the inside of the lower lid on the conjunctiva. Evenly distribute the ointment.
- Have the patient close the eye and gently rub the lid in a circular motion with a cotton ball. This helps distribute the ointment without causing injury to the eye.
- Remove excessive solution or ointment from the lids or face. This promotes comfort and prevents undesired absorption of the medication.
- If ordered by the physician, apply a clean eye patch.

Administering Otic Medications

Task Standard

The perioperative nurse administers otic medications in a manner that
- Prevents injury to the ear
- Maintains the sterility of the medicine dropper
- Prevents the transmission of infection

Purpose of Otic Instillation
- Prevention or treatment of inflammation, discomfort, or infection
- Softening of cerumen for removal

Supplies and Equipment
- Desired otic solution or suspension
- Cotton ball or wick
- Cotton-tipped applicator

Assessing the Patient
- Inspect the site of application for reddened areas, signs of infection, breaks in the skin, and cerumen buildup.

Preparing the Patient
- Position the patient in a comfortable sitting or side-lying position so that the affected ear is facing up. An infant or child can be held by the parent or another adult.
- If cerumen or drainage occludes the outer ear canal, clean the canal with a cotton-tipped applicator. Do not force the cerumen inward or occlude the canal in any way.
- Straighten the adult patient's ear by pulling the pinna upward and outward. For children, pull the pinna down and back. Straightening the canal provides direct access to deeper ear structures.

Instilling the Medication
- Instill the medication by holding the dropper 1 cm above the ear canal. Do not force the drops into the canal under pressure.
- Have the patient maintain the body position for 2 to 3 minutes while applying gentle pressure to the tragus. This allows complete distribution of the solution. Gentle pressure moves the medication inward.
- Insert a cotton ball or wick into the ear (optional). This prevents the solution from running out of the ear when the patient moves the head. Remember to remove the cotton ball.

PHYSIOLOGICALLY MONITORING THE PATIENT

The perioperative nurse demonstrates competency to perform physiologic monitoring of the patient by evaluating
- The airway
- Intake
- Output
- Body temperature
- The effects of local anesthesia

Routine Methods of Monitoring (Table 17)
Monitoring the Airway
Factors That Affect Airway Clearance

- Excessive secretions
- Coexisting respiratory disease
- Tracheostomy
- Obesity
- Fatigue
- Weight of drapes
- Noxious odors
- Flow of blood or secretions into the airway
- Use of medications that produce sedation
- Body position
- Mechanical restriction or reduced ability of the diaphragm to push down against the abdominal contents can impair lung expansion. Lung compliance is then decreased, reducing the

TABLE **17**

Routine Methods of Monitoring

Airway Patency, Gas Exchange, and Tissue Perfusion
Use pulse oximetry
Inspect the skin and nails for color and capillary refill
Inspect the surgical field for color of tissue and blood
Listen to lung sounds and ventilatory rate
Monitor arterial blood gas values as needed

Hemodynamic Status
Assess blood pressure and pulse (rate, rhythm, and quality)
Note the amount and rate of blood loss

Fluid Intake
Inspect mucous membranes and conjunctiva for color, moisture, and edema
Monitor intravenous fluids and blood products
Note the amount and type of surgical irrigation used

Output and Fluid Loss
Assess blood loss, urine output, and other drainage
Assess for third-space fluid loss and insensible fluid loss

Body Temperature
Assess skin temperature and core temperature as needed

Effects of Local Anesthesia
Inspect the skin for rash, edema, or pruritus
Note changes in hemodynamic status, respiratory function, and mental and neurologic status (seizure activity)

amount of alveolar volume available for gas exchange and the functional residual capacity.

Supplies and Equipment

- Nasal cannula or face mask
- Oropharyngeal or nasopharyngeal airway
- Pulse oximeter
- Oxygen
- Endotracheal tube, laryngoscope, self-inflating bag, and pressure-controlled ventilator
- Suction equipment

Preventing Ineffective Airway Clearance

PREOPERATIVE INTERVENTIONS

- Interview the patient and the family to assess for a history of airway obstruction or respiratory disease.
- Conduct an assessment and note the presence of a cough, dyspnea, rales, clubbing of the fingers, abnormal breath sounds, a change in the rate or depth of respiration, and cyanosis.
- Review related laboratory studies:
  1. X-ray film of chest
  2. Sputum studies
  3. Pulmonary function tests
  4. Arterial blood gas studies

INTRAOPERATIVE INTERVENTIONS

- Administer oxygen as needed by means of nasal prongs or a face mask.
- Use a pulse oximeter to determine the blood oxygen saturation.
- Position the patient with the head slightly elevated or in a semi-sitting position if permitted by the surgical procedure.
- Provide emotional support by maintaining contact through touch and communication.
- Monitor the respiratory rate and the quality of chest excursion. Note stridor, change in skin color, or change in mental alertness or personality.
- Observe for signs of airway obstruction:
  1. Inspiration will cause drawing in of parts of the upper chest, the sternum, and the intercostal spaces.
  2. Exhalation is characterized by jerky protrusion and prolonged contractions of abdominal muscles.
  3. Seesaw movement of the chest and abdomen may occur.
  4. Tracheal tug or indrawing of the suprasternal notch may occur.
- Initiate corrective action if airway obstruction occurs.
  1. Open and inspect the mouth for displacement of the tongue and the presence of secretions, blood, or other substances.

2. Extend the head by lifting the patient's jaw. This increases the distance between the chin and the cervical spine, which puts the muscles that support the chin under tension and pulls the tongue forward. This maneuver puts further tension on the musculature that supports the tongue. The mandible is lifted upward by exertion of pressure on the ascending ramus of the mandible and at the same time the head is tilted backward. The fingers and palm of each hand are applied on each side of the face to maintain head extension.

- If the head tilt or extension is not effective, an oral airway may need to be inserted or endotracheal intubation may have to be performed. The perioperative nurse should call for assistance from an anesthetist while administering supplemental oxygen and assisting with ventilation involving use of a self-inflating bag.
- Record findings and report as needed.

POSTOPERATIVE INTERVENTIONS

- Report intraoperative events to the postanesthesia care unit (PACU) or unit nurse.
- Determine the immediate response to therapeutic measures.
- If needed, consult with a respiratory therapist for assistance.

Monitoring Intake

Factors That Affect Fluid and Electrolyte Balance

- Fluid and food intake
- Excessive thirst
- Sources of fluid loss such as diarrhea, draining wounds, excessive urine output, and excessive perspiration
- Use of prescribed medications, such as diuretics and adrenocorticosteroids, that may cause fluid and electrolyte imbalances
- Use of over-the-counter agents to induce urinary and bowel elimination
- Excessive ingestion of alcohol or the use of illegal drugs that may interfere with a proper nutrition
- Preexisting conditions or disease states that can result in fluid and electrolyte imbalances such as diabetes, renal failure, cancer, burns or trauma, and exposure to toxic agents.
- Inadequate IV fluid flow.

Calculating Fluid Need and Flow Rate

$$\frac{\text{Amount of solution to infuse}}{\text{Hours to infuse the solution}} = \text{amount to infuse each hour}$$

or

$$\frac{\text{Amount of solution/hour} \times \text{drops/ml}}{60 \text{ (minutes/hour)}} = \text{drops to infuse/minute}$$

Types of Intravenous Solutions

- Isotonic
  1. Have a total osmolality close to that of intravascular fluid and do not cause red blood cells to shrink or swell.
  2. Commonly used isotonic fluids include 5% dextrose in water, normal saline solution (0.9% sodium chloride), and lactated Ringer solution.
- Hypotonic
  1. Used to replace transcellular fluid because they are hypotonic as compared with plasma.
  2. Commonly used hypotonic fluids include half-normal saline solution (0.45% sodium chloride) and fructose-electrolyte solution (Normosol-M).
- Hypertonic
  1. Have a total osmolality that exceeds that of extracellular fluid.
  2. Commonly used hypertonic solutions include 5% dextrose in normal saline solution (0.9% sodium chloride), dextrose-electrolyte solution (Ionosol MB with 5% dextrose), and hypertonic saline solution (3% sodium chloride).

Infusion Pumps

- Syringe infusion pump
  1. A small pump that may be worn by the patient.
  2. Used to deliver a small volume of solution during a 24-hour period.
- Peristaltic infusion pump
  1. A large infusion pump with a sensor that attaches to any standard IV drip chamber.
  2. Regulates the rate of solution by exerting pressure on the IV tubing and monitors drops per minute infused.
- Piston infusion pump
  1. A large pump that controls solution flow rate by piston action.
  2. Monitors actual volume of fluid infused.

SUPPLIES AND EQUIPMENT
- IV fluid as ordered by the physician
- Venipuncture cannulas
  1. Steel scalp vein needle (butterfly)
  2. Indwelling plastic catheters inserted over a steel needle
  3. Indwelling plastic catheters inserted through a sterile needle
- Tubing
- Infusion pump

Preventing Local Infiltration of IV Fluid

PREOPERATIVE INTERVENTIONS
- Interview the patient or family members and assess for a history of infiltration or problems associated with IV infusion.

- Assess for disease that may alter vascular integrity.
- Select an optimal site for IV entry.
- Upper extremity veins are commonly used.
- Avoid the antecubital fossa because flexion of the arm can impede the flow of the infusion. Select a site that does not impede mobility.
- Use the patient's nondominant hand.
- Palpate the vein for elasticity and the absence of hard knots that may indicate thromboses.

INTRAOPERATIVE INTERVENTIONS

- Frequently inspect the infusion site for infiltration, swelling, redness, or coolness.
- If infiltration occurs, alert the physician. The infusion should be discontinued and restarted.
- Apply a warm, moist compress to the affected area.
- Explain to the patient what has occurred and provide support as needed.
- Record and report care and the patient's response to therapy.

POSTOPERATIVE INTERVENTIONS

- Report intraoperative events to the PACU or unit nurse.
- Determine the immediate response to interventions.

Preventing Fluid Volume Excess

PREOPERATIVE INTERVENTIONS

- Obtain a nursing history and assess the patient for the presence of disease conditions that may put him or her at risk for volume overload.
- Assess baseline laboratory values.
- If the patient is at high risk for hypervolemia, use microdrip tubing and an infusion pump to assist in monitoring intake.
- Note the presence of edema, bounding pulse, distended neck veins, rales, dyspnea, orthopnea, elevated central venous pressure, and recent unexplained weight gain.

INTRAOPERATIVE INTERVENTIONS

- If symptoms of fluid excess develop, slow the rate of the infusion at once and alert the physician.
- Continue to monitor vital signs and report findings to the physician.
- Document findings on the intraoperative record.
- Measure and document urine and blood loss.
- Record and report patient care and response to therapy.

POSTOPERATIVE INTERVENTIONS

- Report intraoperative events to the PACU or unit nurse.
- Determine the immediate response to interventions.

Preventing Air Embolus From IV Catheters

PREOPERATIVE INTERVENTIONS
- Inspect the tubing for the presence of air.
- Flush air from the tubing before connecting it to the patient. Discontinue or replace the infusion before the container is empty.
- Ensure that all connections are tight.

INTRAOPERATIVE INTERVENTIONS
- Allow a loop of tubing to drop below the extremity as an added precaution against air embolus.
- If an air embolus is suspected, clamp the tubing, turn the patient onto the left side, and place the patient in the Trendelenburg position.
- Administer oxygen if an air embolus is suspected and support the circulation with emergency medications as ordered by the physician.
- Record and report intraoperative events, patient care, and the patient's response to care.

POSTOPERATIVE INTERVENTIONS
- Report intraoperative events to the PACU or unit nurse.
- Determine the immediate response to interventions.

Monitoring Output

Factors That Affect Output
- Coexisting disease such as renal failure, neurogenic bladder, urinary retention or diabetes, which can alter normal urine output
- Clotting disorders or the presence of medications in the system that alter normal blood coagulation
- Extremes of age and weight
- Diarrhea
- Artificial urinary drainage system (cystostomy, peritoneal or renal dialysis, ureteral stents)
- Type of surgical procedure, its length and location, and size of the incision
- Trauma
- Use of blood, blood products, IV fluids, and volume expanders

Supplies and Equipment
- Suction tubing and containers
- Sponges
- Graduated measuring devices
- Sterile skin marker and paper for recording the amount of irrigation used

Monitoring Intraoperative Bleeding

PREOPERATIVE INTERVENTIONS

- Conduct an assessment and evaluate for the presence of disease, bleeding or clotting disorders, or medications that may influence blood loss during surgery.
- Assess for the presence of fluid deficit by evaluation of the nutritional status and skin turgor and auscultation of lung field for abnormal breath sounds. Note the presence of medications that may alter fluid balance (IV fluids, bowel preparations, and diuretics).
- Note a family history of bleeding or clotting disorders.
- Start an IV infusion to provide access to the circulatory system.
- Monitor vital signs.

INTRAOPERATIVE INTERVENTIONS

- Prepare and administer IV fluids as needed.
- Insert an indwelling urinary catheter, depending on the patient's fluid status, the anticipated length of the procedure, and the anticipated amount of blood loss.
- Monitor blood loss and the amount of irrigation solution used. Use warm, moistened sponges to prevent tissue from becoming dry and from losing heat via evaporation and convection.
- If the patient is awake, provide psychosocial support during the procedure by using touch, conversation, and measures to distract the patient. Keep blood-soaked sponges and soiled instruments and supplies out of the patient's visual field.
- If hypotension occurs, place the patient in the Trendelenburg position.
- Administer oxygen, fluids, and medications as needed.
- Call for emergency assistance if needed.
- Inspect the wound for a bleeding site if it has not already been located.
- Continue to monitor vital signs.
- Monitor blood loss via suction and saturation of sponges. Weigh sponges as needed.
- Record the type and amount of irrigation fluid used during the procedure.
- Record and report intraoperative care and response to therapy.

POSTOPERATIVE INTERVENTIONS

- Report intraoperative events to the PACU or unit nurse. Communicate estimated blood loss, amount of IV fluid infused, number or units of blood or blood products transfused, and the presence of drains and catheters.
- Determine the immediate response to interventions.

Monitoring Body Temperature
Factors That Affect Body Temperature

- Hypothalamus
- Age and weight
- Activity level
- Inactivity decreases the temperature, whereas vigorous activity may cause an increase.
- Metabolic rate
- Radiation, convection, evaporation, and conduction

Supplies and Equipment

- Thermometer (conventional, electronic, or temperature-sensitive patch or tape)
- Warm blankets
- Fluid warmer
- Hyperthermia or hypothermia blanket and machine

Preventing Hypothermia

PREOPERATIVE INTERVENTIONS

- Interview the patient and family members to assess for factors that may put the patient at risk for hypothermia.
- Wrap the patient in warm sheets or blankets, if needed, while he or she is in the surgical suite holding area.
- Note the preoperative temperature.

INTRAOPERATIVE INTERVENTIONS

- Monitor the patient's temperature and assess physiologic changes.
- Use measures to maintain comfort and warmth.
  1. Increase the ambient temperature of the room.
  2. Provide surface warming with a heating blanket.
  3. Wrap the patient in warm blankets.
  4. Wrap limbs in stockinet, elastic (Ace) wraps, or Webril.
  5. Use warm IV fluids or blood products.
  6. Humidify inspired gases and oxygen.
- Monitor vital signs and note changes in the electrocardiogram, blood pressure, arterial blood gas values, and blood chemistry values.
- Monitor a change in behavior in the awake patient.
- If body temperature drops below the desired level, rewarm the patient as needed. If the temperature is greater than 35°C, passive rewarming is preferred to active rewarming because the latter method may result in hyperthermia. Warming methods include
  1. internal surface warming with warm saline solution, moist sponges, and warm IV fluids

2. external surface warming with a warming blanket, warm sheets, and external packs
- Be prepared for emergency measures, which may include
  1. Cardiac massage (external or internal)
  2. Mechanical ventilation
  3. Infusion of IV fluids and blood products
  4. Cardioversion for ventricular fibrillation
  5. Use of antiarrhythmic drugs
  6. Insertion of an indwelling catheter to monitor fluid status
- Record and report intraoperative findings and care activities.

POSTOPERATIVE INTERVENTIONS
- Report intraoperative events to the PACU or unit nurse.
- Determine the immediate response to interventions.
- Alert the PACU or unit staff to the need for special warming equipment and medications. A number of medications may be used to suppress shivering, including nondepolarizing muscle relaxants in the intubated patient, chlorpromazine, droperidol, magnesium sulfate, and methylphenidate (Miller, 1986, p. 2014).

Preventing Hyperthermia

PREOPERATIVE INTERVENTIONS
- Interview the patient and family members and assess for factors that may put the patient at risk for hyperthermia.
- Note the presence of fever, infection, or diseases associated with hyperthermia.

INTRAOPERATIVE INTERVENTIONS
- Use a thermometer to monitor the patient's temperature and assess changes as needed.
- Maintain the patient's comfort and normal body temperature by removing excessive drapes as needed.
- Cool the patient's skin with alcohol or cool water as needed.
- Monitor vital signs and note changes in the electrocardiogram, blood pressure, arterial blood gas values, and blood chemistry values.
- If body temperature increases, use a cooling blanket as needed. Be prepared for emergency measures, including the use of oxygen, the infusion of cool IV fluids, the use of emergency medications, the use of antiarrhythmic drugs, and the insertion of an indwelling urinary catheter to monitor fluid status.
- Record and report intraoperative findings and care activities.

POSTOPERATIVE INTERVENTIONS
- Report intraoperative events to the PACU or unit nurse.
- Determine the immediate response to interventions.
- Alert the staff of the need for special equipment or medications (e.g., antibiotics and antipyretics).

Monitoring the Effects of Local Anesthesia
Supplies and Equipment

- Local anesthetic agents
- Marker and labels to identify the anesthetic agent on the sterile field
- IV therapy supplies and equipment
- Blood pressure monitor
- Electrocardiographic monitor
- Pulse oximeter
- Emergency supplies
- Oxygen with self-inflating bag and mask
- Endotracheal tube and laryngoscope
- Medications such as diazepam or ultrashort-acting barbiturates such as sodium thiopental, methohexital (Brevital) sodium
- Resuscitative agents

Preventing Extravasation of IV Medication

PREOPERATIVE INTERVENTIONS

- Assess the patient for a history of a local reaction to IV medication.
- Ensure that the IV catheter is patent and flowing before the administration of medication.

INTRAOPERATIVE INTERVENTIONS

- Consult accompanying drug information and related literature before the administration of medication.
- Administer diazepam (Valium).
  1. Do not mix or dilute with other drugs or solutions in the same syringe or container.
  2. Inject slowly, taking at least 1 minute for each 5 mg (1 ml) given to adults and taking 3 minutes to inject 0.25 mg/kg of body weight in children.
  3. Avoid using small veins for diazepam administration.
- Administer midazolam hydrochloride (Versed).
  1. Midazolam injection is compatible with 5% dextrose in water, 0.9% sodium chloride, and lactated Ringer solution.
  2. When midazolam is used for sedation, the perioperative nurse must individualize and titrate the dose. Do not administer midazolam hydrochloride by rapid or single-bolus IV administration. The patient's response varies with age, physical status, and concomitant medication.
- Communicate and record the type of medication administered, the dose, the route, the time of administration, and any local reaction to IV medication.

POSTOPERATIVE INTERVENTIONS

- Report intraoperative events to the PACU or unit nurse.

- Determine the immediate response to interventions.
- Assess postoperative response to local anesthetic agent.

Preventing Cardiodepression Related to the Administration of Local Anesthetics

PREOPERATIVE INTERVENTIONS
- Assess the patient for cardiac disease or the presence of risk factors for cardiac disease. Note drug allergies.
- Establish physiologic baseline values to assess cardiac function during the procedure.

INTRAOPERATIVE INTERVENTIONS
- Monitor the patient. Evaluate
  1. Blood pressure
  2. Heart rate and rhythm
  3. Respiratory rate
  4. Oxygen saturation
  5. Skin condition
  6. Mental status
  7. Emotional response to surgery and anesthesia
- Record and report findings.
- Document at 5-minute intervals and at any significant event.
- Document the dosage, the route and time of administration, and the effect of medications administered, oxygen therapy, and IV therapy and the patient's response to the surgery and anesthesia.

POSTOPERATIVE INTERVENTIONS
- Report intraoperative events to the PACU or unit nurse.
- Determine the immediate response to interventions.

Preventing Ineffective Breathing Pattern Related to IV Sedation

PREOPERATIVE INTERVENTIONS
- Assess the patient for a history of sensitivity to sedatives and narcotics.
- Assess for signs of pulmonary dysfunction: dyspnea, tachypnea, orthopnea, skin color changes, absent or diminished breath sounds, rhonchi, wheezing, or rales.
- Establish physiologic baseline values to assess respiratory function during the procedure.
- Note the patient's weight and calculate the maximal dosage.
- Note reports of respiratory status tests (chest x-ray films, pulmonary function tests).

INTRAOPERATIVE INTERVENTIONS
- Position the patient to facilitate breathing. Elevate the head and ensure that drapes and equipment are kept off the chest if possible.

- As ordered by the physician, provide humidified oxygen at the desired rate (liters per minute).
- Monitor the patient. Evaluate
  1. Blood pressure
  2. Heart rate and rhythm
  3. Respiratory rate
  4. Oxygen saturation
  5. Skin condition
  6. Mental status
  7. Emotional response to surgery and anesthesia
- Record and report findings.
- Document at 5-minute intervals and at any significant event.
- Document the dosage, the route and time of administration, the effect of medications administered, oxygen therapy, and IV therapy, and the patient's response to the surgery and anesthesia.

POSTOPERATIVE INTERVENTIONS

- Report intraoperative events to the PACU or unit nurse.
- Determine the immediate response to interventions.

MONITORING AND CONTROLLING THE ENVIRONMENT

The perioperative nurse demonstrates competency to monitor and control the environment by

- Regulating temperature and humidity
- Ensuring electrical safety
- Monitoring the sensory environment
- Ensuring radiation safety
- Maintaining surgical suite traffic patterns
- Performing operating room (OR) sanitation
- Sterilizing instruments, supplies, and equipment

Regulating Temperature and Humidity

- The perioperative nurse is responsible for monitoring room temperature and humidity levels.
- A relative humidity of 50% to 60% inhibits bacterial growth and decreases the potential for static electricity.
- Room temperatures of 68°F to 76°F inhibit bacterial growth.

Supplies and Equipment

- Devices for monitoring room temperature and humidity
- Overhead warming units
- Heat conduction lamps
- Cooling or warming blankets
- Blood warmers
- Thermal body drapes

- Cloth blankets
- Warming cabinets for solutions and blankets
- Patient temperature–monitoring devices
  1. Esophageal
  2. Urinary bladder
  3. Axillary
  4. Rectal
  5. Tympanic

Monitoring the Temperature and Humidity of the Operating Room

- Before starting the first case of the day, take a baseline reading of the OR temperature and humidity level. The temperature should range between 68°F and 76°F. The humidity level should range between 50% and 60%.
- Report variations of these ranges to the OR manager.
- Except in extenuating circumstances, such as an emergency situation or when the room temperature is raised to accommodate a patient at risk for alteration in body temperature, avoid using ORs that do not adhere to these ranges.

Assessing the Need for Devices to Monitor and/or Control the Patient's Temperature

- Consider the following factors when assessing the patient for temperature monitoring and/or control devices:
  1. The patient's age
  2. The patient's physical status
  3. Type of anesthesia planned
  4. Ambient room temperature
  5. Length and type of surgical procedure (AORN, 1992, *III*:7–2)

Monitoring the Temperature of the Patient

- Use a thermometer with an appropriate esophageal, urinary bladder, tympanic, axillary, or rectal probe to monitor patients at risk for experiencing intraoperative alterations in body temperature.
- Before using the thermometer, test it according to the manufacturer's instructions to ensure that it is in working order.
- After obtaining the desired probe, carefully insert it into the appropriate orifice.
- Insert probes after the patient is anesthetized for easier insertion, protection of the patient's dignity, and to avoid adverse affects such as vagal stimulation with the rectal probe.
- Place the rectal probe in the adult patient; insert it 1 to 2 inches within the rectum.
- For the infant, insert the rectal probe no more than 1 inch.
- Gently insert tympanic membrane probes.

- After inserting a probe, tape it into place to avoid inadvertent removal during the procedure.

Conserving the Patient's Body Heat
- Conserve the patient's body heat by covering the patient with warm blankets.
- Expose only the operative area.
- Decrease air currents by keeping the OR doors closed and limiting movement within the OR.
- Warm preparation solutions, intravenous infusions, blood, and irrigating solutions.
- Moisten sponges with warm saline solution before handing them to the surgeon.
- Keep the OR bed linens dry.
- Blot the patient's skin dry after the skin preparation.

Alternative Methods of Temperature Regulation
- Provide thermoregulation devices such as warming or cooling blankets and heat lamps for patients identified as being at high risk for alterations in body temperature.

Neonates
- The neonate, especially during the first 24 hours of life, is at risk for experiencing an intraoperative alteration in body temperature.
- Conserve the neonate's body heat by covering the head with a stockinet cap, encasing the extremities in stockinet, or wrapping the extremities with Webril or plastic wrap.
- Use warming blankets and heat lamps. Exercise caution when employing these devices because the thin layer of subcutaneous fat places the neonate at risk for experiencing a thermal injury.
- Keep the neonate in an Isolette and dressed before and immediately after the procedure to conserve the patient's body heat.

Documentation Procedures
- Document the use of thermoregulation devices and skin conditions before and after the procedure.
- Record the patient's baseline temperature. This helps in the detection of malignant hyperthermia and overheating from auxiliary heating equipment.

Ensuring Electrical Safety
Monitoring Isolated Power Systems for Effectiveness
- The OR isolated power system prevents accidental grounding of persons in contact with a hot wire.
- The isolated power system continually monitors for current leaks and grounding and thus reduces the hazard of shock, cardiac fib-

rillation, or burns from electrical current flowing through the patient's body to ground (AORN, 1992, *III:7–4*).

- If the isolated power system is functional, the alarm sounds only when faulty equipment is plugged into ungrounded circuits. In such a case, shut off and unplug the last electrical device plugged into the electrical system.
- If the warning system alarm light remains on, unplug electrical equipment until the defective device is identified.
- After the defective device is found, send it to the bioengineering department for repair.

Providing Safe Electrical Equipment

- Ensure that all electrical equipment, including the surgeon's personal equipment, meets hospital performance and safety standards.
- Ensure that routine inspections occur at least every 6 months to check for defects. Schedule preventive maintenance in accordance with manufacturer's recommendations to prolong equipment life and enhance patient safety.
- Before using electrical equipment for patient care, inspect the equipment for frayed cords, loose wires, and lack of secure connections.
- Test the electrical units before use for functioning audio alarms and lights.
- Check outlets and switch plates for damage (AORN, 1992, *III:7–4*).
- Do not use equipment that requires unusually high-power settings to function. Turn this equipment in for repair.
- Test electrical adapters for tightness to ensure a secure connection. If necessary, replace the adapter.

Implementing Electrical Safety Practices

- Do not place receptacles containing liquid on top of electrical equipment. Inadvertent spills may ruin the equipment and injure the patient and staff members.
- During cleaning procedures, avoid saturating electrical equipment with liquid.
- Do not spray liquid directly onto equipment; clean with a damp cloth.
- During the procedure, ensure that foot pedals that activate electrical equipment remain dry.
- Do not roll heavy equipment (beds, x-ray machines) over electrical cords.
- Position equipment during procedures to decrease stress on electrical cords and connections.

- Avoid using extension cords. If extension cords are necessary, use only those that are designed for heavy-duty use and approved by the hospital biomedical engineering department.
- Replace short cords of high-use equipment with long cords.
- Maintain a safe traffic pattern by taping electrical cords securely to the floor. When removing cords from sockets, do not pull on the wire; remove by the plug.

Monitoring the Sensory Environment
Supplies and Equipment
- Audio equipment
- Air freshener devices
- Air filtration devices
- Screens

Providing Preoperative Teaching
- Fear and anxiety, common reactions in many surgical patients, are often related to knowledge deficit.
- Use preoperative teaching to confirm expectations and clarify misconceptions concerning the surgical experience.
- Begin the preoperative teaching by assessing the patient's knowledge level about the surgical environment.
- Clarify misconceptions and explain what to expect in the surgical suite.
- Tell the patient about environmental sights, sounds, and smells.

Eliminating, Attenuating, and Modifying Sensory Stimuli
- Establish traffic patterns so that the patient avoids areas where noxious sights, sounds, or smells occur.
- Place the patient in an area that shields him or her from distressing stimuli.
- If the patient has a local, regional, or spinal anesthetic, arrange the drapes and screen to prevent visualization of the procedure, blood, specimens, instruments, and equipment.
- Keep loud talking to a minimum.
- Monitor conversations and exercise caution when using the intercommunication system.
- Do not talk during the induction of general anesthesia.
- Handle instruments quietly in the presence of the patient.
- When testing or using noisy instruments and equipment (drills, saws, alarms, laminar air flow equipment), warn the patient and explain what to expect.
- If surgery generates noxious odors, explain these to the conscious patient.
- Use music to distract the conscious patient during surgery.

- Provide diversionary activities when appropriate.
- Use coached breathing exercises and guided imagery to distract the patient.
- Use touch and verbal reassurance to comfort the patient and thus possibly reduce anxiety and fear.

Ensuring Radiation Safety
Supplies and Equipment

- Radiation exposure badges or monitoring devices
- Lead aprons
- Lead gloves
- Lead collars and shields
- X-ray cassette–holding devices
- Portable or stationary x-ray equipment

Monitoring the Amount of Radiation Exposure

- The OR manager provides radiation-monitoring badges for personnel frequently exposed to ionizing radiation.
- Wear badges outside lead aprons at the neckline and ring dosimeters when the hands are exposed to radiation.
- If pregnant, avoid radiation exposure.

Providing Protective Devices

- Before use, inspect leaded protective devices for cracks.
- Biannually, the OR manager should have leaded protective devices radiographically inspected for cracks and structural integrity.
- Provide lead gloves to personnel who must hold the x-ray cassette while x-ray films are taken; this protects their hands.
- Wear lead aprons to protect the torso and gonads.
- Wear lead collars to protect the thyroid.
- During upper torso exposure of the male patient, place a lead collar over the testicles.
- During x-ray exposures, the surgical team should move as far away from the radiation source as possible.
- Protect the staff who cannot leave the room by placing a portable lead shield on a movable stand in a convenient location in the OR.
- Drape shields adjacent to the sterile field with sterile sheets.
- After use, store leaded protective devices flat or hanging, never folded.

Implementing Radioactive Material Safety Precautions

- The perioperative nurse coordinates the intraoperative insertion of radioactive materials (seeds, needles, capsules).

- Nuclear medicine personnel transport radioactive material to the OR.
- Store the carrier for radioactive implants away from personnel and patient care areas.
- Identify and document the number of radioactive items when they are delivered to the OR.
- During insertion, stay as far away from the source of radiation as possible.
- Do not touch radioactive material with bare or gloved hands.
- Use the instruments provided for insertion and handling when moving or touching radioactive material.
- Handle radiation material as quickly as possible to limit exposure.
- Before the patient leaves the OR, establish accountability by counting the radioactive material.
- Account for each item implanted and retained in the container.
- After implantation of radioactive materials, notify recovery or floor personnel that they will receive a patient with radioactive implants.

Documentation Procedures
- Include in the operative record the type of ionizing radiation used.
- Monitor and record the monthly radiation exposures for personnel.
- Document the time, number, location, and types of radioactive material inserted.
- Place a sign indicating that radiation is in use on the door of the OR while the procedure is in progress.
- Inform the postanesthesia care unit or floor personnel before receiving the patient so that they can make arrangements for care of the patient.
- A radiation safety officer should maintain written records of radioactive materials.

Ensuring Laser Safety
Selecting Qualified Personnel for Laser Use
- Physicians, nurses, technicians, and others required to work with lasers must demonstrate competency in laser techniques and have knowledge concerning the hazards of and safety measures for laser surgery.

Providing Safe Laser Units
- When laser equipment is not in use, secure the unit.
- Access to the laser key is limited to personnel qualified in laser use.

- Before each use, and before bringing the patient into the room, check and test the laser equipment.
- Immediately report equipment malfunction, and do not use the unit until it is repaired.
- Closely follow the manufacturer's recommendations and instructions when operating laser equipment.
- Rooms for laser use should not have windows, or the windows should have blinds. Evacuate the laser plume through filtered hospital lines or specific equipment designed for this purpose.
- When the laser equipment is not in immediate use, place it on standby to avoid accidental discharge.

Providing Laser Protective Devices

- When using the laser, place on the door a warning sign that a laser is in use and that protective eyewear is required.
- Ensure that personnel wear approved protective glasses with side shields.
- Cover the eyes of the awake patient with appropriate protective glasses.
- Cover the eyes of anesthetized patients with reflective barrier and tape in place.
- Protect patients and health care workers from inhaling laser fumes.
- Use special nonreflective instruments during laser surgery.
- Laser safety devices
  1. Protective wear specific for laser wavelength
  2. Wet gauze or cloth towels should be used for carbon dioxide wavelength
  3. Special anesthesia endotracheal equipment for head and neck surgery
  4. Nonreflective instruments
  5. Signs indicating that laser surgery is in progress with wavelength, power, and eyewear necessary (AORN, 1992, III:10–1—10–3).

Implementing Fire Safety Precautions

- Since laser beams may ignite flammable supplies such as drapes, gowns, and clothing, do not allow the use of flammable anesthetics.
- Use endotracheal tubes designed for laser use for head and neck procedures.
- Ensure that skin preparation solutions do not have an alcohol base.
- Drape moistened towels around the incision area before laser use.
- Use laser-retardant drapes to drape the operative site.

- Keep the towels and sponges surrounding the target tissue wet at all times.
- Have a bucket of water in the room in case flammable materials are ignited.
- Have a halon fire extinguisher readily available during a laser procedure.

Documentation Procedures

- Documentation on the operative record includes
  1. Name of the surgeon
  2. Support staff
  3. Procedure
  4. Type of laser used
  5. Lens used
  6. Length of laser use
  7. Wattage
- Additional laser logs may be required by the institution or the U.S. Food and Drug Administration if equipment is listed as investigational.
- Document orientation and ongoing education programs for nursing personnel performing laser procedures. Post warning signs indicating laser use.

Maintaining Traffic Patterns

Traffic Pattern Zones

- The unrestricted zone includes the areas where OR personnel interface with outside departments, the patient reception and holding areas, and areas where supplies are received. In some surgical suites, the unrestricted zone also includes communication stations and administrative offices. Personnel may wear street clothes in the unrestricted zone.
- The semirestricted zone may include, but is not limited to, storage and instrument-processing areas and, depending on design, corridors leading to restricted areas and peripheral support areas. Personnel must don appropriate scrub attire to enter the semirestricted zone.
- In the restricted zone, personnel must wear appropriate scrub attire and surgical masks. This area includes the ORs, substerile areas, and the sterile core areas.

Supplies and Equipment

- Scrub attire
- Masks
- Hair covering
- Shoe covers

- Germicidal solutions for cleaning
- Personal protective attire (eyewear, gloves, aprons)
- Enclosed transport carts for contaminated items

Decreasing Potential Airborne Contamination

- Keep traffic flow into and out of the room to a minimum.
- Because corridor air may contain a higher bacterial count than OR air, keep doors closed. Open doors only when transporting patients, supplies, or equipment (AORN, 1992, *III:22–2*).
- Bar sick personnel, or those with skin infections, from working in restricted areas.

Decreasing Potential Contamination From Outside Environmental Sources

- Before use, damp dust or wipe down with a germicidal solution all equipment brought into the surgical suite.
- Transport clean and sterile items to the OR in an enclosed container or on a covered cart.
- Before bringing supply carts into the OR, remove protective coverings.
- Clean patient-transport gurneys after each use (AORN, 1992, *III:17–3*).

Confining Contamination Within Established Traffic Patterns

- Contain contamination by transporting trash, soiled linen, soiled instruments, and nonsterile equipment and supplies in an enclosed cart or an impervious system.
- Ensure that contaminated objects and waste-disposal operations are separate from patient care areas.
- Contain contaminated items at the source or origin to decrease airborne contamination (AORN, 1992, *III:17–2*).

Providing Clear Pathways for Traffic Flow

- To facilitate retrieval and traffic patterns, store supplies as close as possible to their point of use.
- Keep hallways free of clutter to decrease potential injury and ease the flow of traffic.
- When carts and equipment must be in hallways, keep them isolated to one side of the hallway so there is an aisle for traffic flow.

Performing Operating Room Sanitation
General Principles

- Every surgical procedure is considered potentially contaminated.
- Implement the same environmental sanitation protocols for every surgical procedure (AORN, 1992, *III:17–1*).

- Closely follow Universal precautions, as designated by the Centers for Disease Control (CDC) during all environmental sanitation procedures.
- Sanitation measures are required before, during, and after each procedure.

Supplies and Equipment
- Lint-free cloths for cleaning
- Germicidal solutions
- Wet vacuum (preferred) or a mop and clean mop heads
- Mechanical floor scrubber
- Plastic liners
- Gloves
- Pistol-grip sprayer
- Laundry bags
- Disposable suction tubing
- Suction containers
- Utility carts
- Covered carts for linens and trash disposal

Personnel Protection
- Personnel with exudative lesions or weeping dermatitis should not perform environmental sanitation duties.
- Use protective devices such as gloves, gowns, masks, protective eyewear, and instruments when handling contaminated articles.

Preoperative Sanitation
- Before the first scheduled surgery, damp dust all horizontal surfaces, including furniture, surgical lights, and equipment, with a clean, lint-free cloth moistened in a hospital-grade disinfectant.
- Use friction while damp-dusting.
- For subsequent procedures, perform preoperative sanitation by inspecting the room for cleanliness. If discrepancies are found, make corrections before preparing the room for the next procedure. If additional equipment is needed for the next procedure, damp dust the equipment before bringing it into the room (AORN, 1992, *III*:17–3).

Intraoperative Sanitation
- During the surgical procedure confine and contain contamination to a small area.
- Use appropriate protective devices (gloves, instruments, eyewear, gowns) when handling contaminated articles.
- When organic debris falls from the sterile field, remove with a disposable cloth and promptly disinfect the area.

- Saturate the area with a germicidal solution and wipe with a clean cloth. Discard the contaminated cloth into an impervious container.
- Deposit soiled sponges in a plastic-lined bucket.
- Do not place soiled sponges on a draped table or spread on an impervious barrier on the floor.
- If the anesthetist must see the sponges, ask her or him to stand up and look or take the bucket to the anesthetist.
- When necessary, count sponges and seal them in an impervious bag (AORN, 1992, *III*:19–2).
- While wearing gloves, pick up surgical instruments that fall on the floor and submerge them in a pan containing germicidal detergent. This prevents drying of debris, which would become airborne contamination.
- Enclose nonsubmersible instruments in a clean impervious container, such as a plastic bag or case cart.
- If contaminated instruments are required for immediate use, before sterilization, wash in a germicidal detergent and rinse.
- Clean the exterior surfaces of impervious specimen containers received from the operative field with a disinfectant before attaching a label and removing from the OR.
- Ensure that documents submitted with specimens are free from contamination. Identify and label specimens as contaminated (AORN, 1992, *III*:17–2).

Postoperative Sanitation

- At the end of the procedure, clean with germicidal solution all horizontal surfaces and surfaces that have come in immediate contact with a patient or patient secretions.
- Disconnect disposable suction units, seal, and discard.
- If hospital policy dictates disposal of suction container fluids, empty contents of the suction container into a flushing hopper.
- Use protective eyewear, masks or face shield, apron or gown, and gloves when disposing of suction container fluids.
- If a reusable suction container is used, disinfect after each use (AORN, 1992, *III*:17–2).
- Confine all disposable items used during the procedure in impervious containers.
- Use gloves when handling contaminated linens or trash and handle as little as possible.
- Place all linens, used and unused, in a designated laundry bag.
- Place wet linen in the center of the bag to prevent inadvertent seepage.
- Seal and remove to a designated area trash, linen, and hazardous wastes (AORN, 1992, *III*:17–2).

- Wear gloves when handling items that were on the sterile field or that came in contact with the patient.
- Separate instruments and supplies that were not on the sterile field or in contact with the patient from contaminated items.
- Irrigate suction tips with clean water before disconnecting.
- Remove all visible debris from contaminated instruments and open the jaws of locking instruments.
- Separate delicate instruments for special handling and disassemble instruments that can reasonably be handled without losing parts.
- Place sharps into puncture-proof containers.
- Do not recap needles or disassemble disposable syringes when disposing of sharps.
- Remove blades from knife handles with a needle holder.
- Separate sharp instruments (skin hooks, scissors, rakes, osteotome, towel clips) and place in an appropriate container such as an emesis basin.
- Deposit reusable needles and sharp instruments in a puncture-proof container for transport to a processing area.
- If the substerile area adjacent to the OR contains the washer-sterilizer, place instruments in a wire mesh tray for processing.
- If the processing area is not adjacent to the OR, place contaminated instruments in a plastic bag or enclosed cart for transport.
- Remove gown and gloves before leaving the OR (AORN, 1992, *III*:17–2).
- After removing trash, linen, and instruments, flood the floors with a germicidal detergent and wet-vacuum.
- If a wet vacuum is not available, mop the floor with a clean mop head soaked in fresh germicidal detergent solution.
- After mopping, discard the mop head (AORN, 1992, *III*:17–3).
- When cleaning the OR bed, wipe all surfaces and mattress pads with a lint-free cloth soaked in germicidal detergent. Pay particular attention to the sides of the OR bed.
- If the OR bed was modified for the lithotomy position, inspect and clean the underside of the foot section.
- After thoroughly cleaning the OR bed, move it to the periphery of the OR, thus allowing easy access to the center of the room for wet-vacuuming or mopping.
- When moving the OR bed, move casters of the table through the cleaning solution.
- Carefully inspect the overhead lights for contamination and spot-clean as needed.
- After cleaning, wipe the surgical light reflector shields with 70% isopropyl alcohol to remove detergent film.
- Return the lights to the center of the room for optimum lighting exposure.

- Remove reusable anesthesia tubing, masks, and equipment and deposit for terminal cleaning.
- Discard disposable tubing, masks, endotracheal tubes, and other equipment into trash containers.
- Disinfect horizontal surfaces of the anesthesia machine (AORN, 1992, *III*:1–1).
- Inspect OR walls for contamination and spot clean as necessary (AORN, 1992, *III*:17–3).
- Clean transportation gurneys with germicidal solution after each use. Pay attention to cleaning side rails, mattress, pillows, and any other area that may have been contaminated with blood or body fluids (AORN, 1992, *III*:17–3).
- After the room is cleaned, remove gloves, wash the hands, and prepare the room for the next case by placing new liners and bags in the appropriate receptacles for trash and linen.
- Reassemble the suction canisters and attach clean tubing.
- Prepare the OR bed with fresh linen and a clean safety strap.

Sanitation at the Conclusion of the Scheduled Day

- At the end of each day, terminally clean all ORs, substerile areas, scrub sinks, scrub or utility areas, hallways, furniture, and equipment.
- In sterile storage areas, avoid contaminating sterile supplies with cleaning solutions.
- Remove all portable equipment such as kick buckets, linen hamper frames, suction canisters, and other waste receptacles from the room and clean with a germicidal detergent.
- Autoclave items such as kick buckets that contained body fluids.
- Wipe down overhead lights, doors, handles on cabinets, waste receptacles, and remaining furniture or room equipment.
- Flood the floor with a germicidal detergent for 5 minutes and thoroughly scrub with a floor scrubber.
- Remove the solution with a wet vacuum or a clean, single-use mop head.
- If baseboards are present, use a baseboard brush for cleaning before removing the floor-cleaning solution.
- Disassemble, clean, and, if possible, autoclave reusable soap dispensers before refilling.
- Remove and autoclave spray heads of faucets.
- Inspect walls, particularly around scrub sink areas, for cleanliness.
- Clean transportation and storage carts. After performing OR sanitation, clean the housekeeping equipment.
- Before storing the equipment, ensure that it is dry, because moisture tends to enhance bacterial growth (AORN, 1992, *III*:17–3).

Periodic Sanitation for the Surgical Suite

- Routinely clean cabinets and shelves, walls, the ceiling, air conditioning and heating grills, ducts and filters, sterilizers, warming cabinets, refrigerator, offices, lounges, and locker rooms (AORN, 1992, *III*:17–3).

Sterilizing Instruments, Supplies, and Equipment
Supplies and Equipment

- Gravity displacement autoclave
- Prevacuum autoclave
- Autoclave recording graphs
- Biologic and chemical sterilization indicators
- Ethylene oxide sterilizer
- Ethylene oxide aerator

Decontaminating Instruments
CLEANING

- During the surgical procedure, keep instruments free from gross blood and other debris by wiping or prerinsing with distilled water.
- After the procedure is completed, open used instruments and place in water or a germicidal solution.
- Collect and take used supplies and equipment to the decontamination section of the instrument-processing area in a way that avoids contamination of personnel or any area of the hospital.
- If working in the decontamination area, wear protective clothing, which includes a scrub uniform, a plastic apron or jumpsuit, hair covering, rubber or plastic gloves, and safety glasses.

Delicate Instruments

- Hand-wash delicate instruments with a germicidal detergent that will not damage the instrument. After washing, place the delicate instruments in a wire mesh pan, put in a sterilizer, and sterilize for 3 minutes at 270°F.
- Use a liquid disinfectant for the processing of the hand-washed instruments.
- Thoroughly wash and dry instruments before placing them in the disinfectant. Drying prevents dilution of the disinfectant.
- Take precautions to avoid contact with these chemicals.
- After the disinfection process is complete, rinse the items in distilled water, dry, and store or send to the packaging area for further processing.

General Instruments

- For general instruments, use automated cleaners or washer-sterilizers for decontamination.

- Carefully take instruments from the fluid-filled basins, place in wire mesh trays, and put into the washer-sterilizer for washing, rinsing, and sterilizing.
- If washer-sterilizers are not available, wash the instruments manually.
- When manually cleaning the instruments, submerge them in the appropriate germicidal detergent and clean while they are submerged.

Ultrasonic Cleaning

- After the initial washing of general instruments, place the instruments in an ultrasonic cleaner, which removes debris that may have been missed.
- Do not combine dissimilar metal such as copper, stainless steel, and brass in the ultrasonic cleaner.
- Make sure that all instruments in the ultrasonic baskets are covered with solution.
- After the ultrasonic cycle, drain and rinse instruments.
- Lubricate instruments that have been in the ultrasonic cleaner with a water-soluble solution; this protects the instruments from corrosion and rust and improves the movement of joints.
- Allow water-soluble solutions to dry on the instrument, thereby providing a protective coating.

Preparing Instruments, Equipment, and Supplies for Sterilization

- Inspect instruments for cleanliness and proper functioning before preparing them for sterilization.
- Open the box locks of instruments for the sterilization cycle.
- Ensure that stringers or rack box locks remain open.
- If possible, disassemble instruments with multiple parts before sterilization.
- Place instruments that will be sterilized together in perforated container systems or wire-mesh trays.
- Place heavy instruments in the bottom of the tray.
- Wrap delicate instruments separately and place on top of the heavy instruments.
- To ensure that all surfaces are exposed to the sterilizing agent, place absorbent towels between nested articles.
- Ensure that the weight of instrument sets does not exceed approximately 16 pounds (AORN, 1992, *III*:20–1).
- Before wrapping the instruments, place chemical sterilization indicators in the center of each pack.
- When steam-sterilizing items with lumina, such as tubes, needles, and drains, flush with distilled water before placing them in

the tray. This prevents the trapping of air, thus facilitating the steam sterilization process.
- If ethylene oxide or chemical sterilization processes are used, ensure that lumina are dry.

Wrapping Items
- Use sterilization wrapping materials that permit penetration of the sterilizing agent to all items in the package.
- If using woven materials, ensure that material is freshly laundered.
- Check material for holes or a minimal number of heat-sealed patches.
- Whether using single-use disposable or reusable fabric wrappers, sequentially double wrap the items for sterilization.

Packaging Items
- Ensure that peel-pack pouches have as much air as possible removed before sealing.
- Ensure that like materials of peel-pack pouches touch when double-wrapping (paper to paper, see-through plastic to plastic).
- Ensure that packaging completely covers the item. (AORN, 1992, *III*:12–1—12–2).

Performing Steam Sterilization
Loading Items for Steam Sterilization
- Place each item on the autoclave racks to ensure free circulation of steam.
- If an item capable of holding water, such as basins and solid-bottomed trays, is sterilized, place it on its side during the sterilization cycle.
- Place flat packages on the shelf vertically.
- Place large packages so that they do not touch.
- Place linen packages on the top level of the sterilizer and metal items on the bottom when running a mixed load.
- Place heat-sealed plastic-paper peel-down packages on end. This will keep them upright.
- Instrument-container systems and sets with perforated trays may be placed flat during the sterilization cycle.

Operating a Steam Sterilizer
- Follow the manufacturer's written instructions when operating the steam sterilizer.
- Before removing the contents, check the sterilizer graph or printed readout to verify that sterilization objectives were met.
- When ready to remove the sterilizer contents, before opening the door, verify that the exhaust valve reading is zero to ensure complete dissipation of steam.

TABLE **18**

Minimum Sterilization Exposure Period for Wrapped and Unwrapped Goods: Gravity Cycle Only

Items

Dressings, wrapped in muslin or an equivalent

Glassware, empty, inverted

Instruments, metal combined with suture, tubing, or other porous materials, unwrapped

Instruments, metal only, in mesh-bottomed tray, unwrapped

Instruments, wrapped in double-thickness muslin or an equivalent

Textile packs (maximum size: $12 \times 12 \times 20$ inches; maximum weight: 12 pounds)

Treatment trays, wrapped in muslin or an equivalent

Utensils, wrapped in muslin or an equivalent

Utensils, unwrapped

Flasked solutions

75 ml

250 ml

500 ml

1000 ml

1500 ml

2000 ml

*Dry time for wrapped goods can vary depending on pack density, instrument tray weight, pack-preparation technique including type of wrapping material used, and sterilizer-loading procedures.

†Dry time is not required for unwrapped goods; however, on older sterilizers a dry time of 1 or 2 minutes will help reduce excess steam when opening chamber door at end of cycle.

Adapted with permission from American Sterilizer Company (AMSCO), *Eagle series 3000 equipment manual*, AMSCO publication number P-124362-451 (pp. 12–13) and *Sterilization Guidelines* (1987), p. 5, Erie, Pa.

- Stand behind the door and open it slowly to avoid the steam escaping from around the door.
- Do not touch the interior surfaces of the sterilizer because of the potential for burns.
- Keep the doors of sterilizers closed when not in use.
- Sterilize supplies requiring the same exposure cycle in the same load (Table 18).
- After removing the cart from the sterilizer, do not place it near air vents or fans because of the possibility of condensation.
- Items removed from the sterilizer after processing are kept on the cart until adequately cooled.
- Do not touch sterile items while cooling.
- Consider wet packages unsterile.

Sterilize Times at 250°F (121°C) (Minutes)	Sterilize Times at 270°F (132°C) (Minutes)	Dry Times (Minutes)
30	25	30*
15	3	0†
20	10	0†
15	3	0†
30	15	30*
30	25	30*
30	15	30*
30	15	30*
15	3	0†
	N/A	N/A
25		
30		
40		
45		
50		
55		

- Apply dust covers to designated items after they are completely cooled.

Operating a High-Speed Pressure (Flash) Sterilizer

- Use high-speed, uncovered (flash) sterilization for emergencies only.
- Place unwrapped items in a perforated or mesh-bottomed tray.
- Position instruments that have concave surfaces with the open side down and open all hinged instruments.
- Use racks or stringers to ensure that instruments stay open during sterilization.
- Disassemble items with easily removable parts.
- Separate heavy items from delicate instruments to decrease potential damage.

- Sterilize metal instruments for 3 minutes at or above 270°F.
- Sterilize porous items (towels, rubber or plastic) or mixed porous-nonporous items for 10 minutes at or above 270°F.
- Specialty instruments may require different exposure times based on the manufacturers' recommendations.
- Do not flash-sterilize heat-sensitive items.
- Do not flash-sterilize implants; these require sterilization in conjunction with biologic monitoring.
- Use a sterile device (towels, handles, mittens) for removing instruments from the autoclave.
- Remove instruments by an aseptic technique (AORN, 1992, *III*:20–6).

Sterilizing With Ethylene Oxide
Implementing Safety Procedures
- Operate ethylene oxide sterilizers according to the manufacturer's recommendation and equipment specifications.
- Since ethylene oxide vapor is extremely hazardous, avoid inhaling vapors.
- Isolate all ethylene oxide sterilizers and aerators to minimize human exposure to toxic vapors.
- Do not smoke near ethylene oxide because it is highly flammable and explosive.
- Post signs identifying where ethylene oxide is in use.
- Ensure that persons operating ethylene oxide sterilizers are knowledgeable about chemical hazards and emergency procedures.
- Monitor all personnel who may be potentially exposed to ethylene oxide.

Loading Ethylene Oxide Sterilizers
- Sterilize items that have common aeration times together.
- Thoroughly clean and dry items before sterilization.
- Dry the lumina of tubing and needles to avoid the formation of ethylene glycol from the combination of water and ethylene oxide.
- After packaging the items, place on metal carts or in wire baskets. Avoid overloading the sterilizer. This allows circulation of sterilant to all surfaces.
- Arrange items so that they do not touch the walls of the sterilizing chamber during the sterilizing cycle.
- Do not stack heavy packages on top of one another, and place pouches on edge in a wire basket (AORN, 1992, *III*:20–4—20–5).

Transferring Items From Sterilizer to Aerator
- Open the sterilizer door as soon as possible after completion of the sterilization cycle to decrease ethylene oxide vapor buildup.

- If sterilizer carts are used when moving equipment from the sterilizer to the aerator, pull the carts, do not push them, to avoid inhaling ethylene oxide.
- Avoid touching sterilized items when transferring sterilized items to the aerator because ethylene oxide can burn the skin.
- Use gloves when removing the biologic indicator test pack from the sterilized load and wash the hands to remove any possible gas residue.

Aerating Items

- Leave approximately 1 inch between all items. Overloading the aerator decreases air circulation, which in turn prolongs the aeration cycle.
- Do not open the aerators until the entire cycle time has elapsed.
- Do not remove items from the aerator prematurely.
- At the completion of the cycle, allow items to cool before storage.

Monitoring the Sterilization Process
Mechanical Control Measures

- Monitor mechanical control monitors such as time-temperature recording devices, temperature gauges, and pressure gauges at the beginning and end of each cycle to verify that adequate parameters have been achieved.
- Before removing any materials from the sterilizer, verify that adequate temperature and duration have been achieved.
- Report sterilizer malfunction or suspicious operation to the appropriate person.
- If automated mechanical control measures are used, evaluate and initial the recording at the end of each cycle.

Chemical Indicators

- Use the manufacturer's criteria to interpret chemical indicator results.
- Use an external chemical indicator with every package.
- Place an internal chemical indicator in the most inaccessible area of every pack.

Efficacy of Vacuum System on Prevacuum Sterilizers

- Use the Bowie-Dick test to determine the efficacy of the vacuum system of a prevacuum sterilizer.
- Place a Bowie-Dick type of test sheet in the center of a pack consisting of folded towels, 9 × 12 inches, with a height of 10 to 11 inches. Ensure that the pack is loosely single wrapped.
- Place the test pack horizontally on the bottom front rack of the sterilizer, near the door and over the drain of an otherwise empty chamber.

- Run this test each day before the first sterilization cycle. Do not perform this test on gravity displacement sterilizers.

Biologic Testing of Sterilizers

- Perform biologic testing for routine monitoring and as a challenge test after any major sterilizer redesign or relocation, suspected malfunction, and major repair.
- Perform biologic testing at least weekly or as needed for steam autoclaves.

Procedure

- Label the biologic indicator with sterilizer load information.
- Place the indicator in the area of the sterilizer chamber that is least favorable to sterilization.
- Remove it from the sterilizer after exposure to the sterilization cycle.
- Incubate the biologic indicator according to the manufacturer's recommendations.
- Schedule biologic testing according to institutional policies. At a minimum, biologically test a sterilizer at least weekly.
- Record the results of biologic indicator tests.
- Notify appropriate personnel immediately if abnormal results occur.
- Place biologic indicators in any load that includes implants.
- Do not use the implants until the return of a normal biologic indicator at 48 hours.
- Use *Bacillus stearothermophilus* to test steam sterilization and *B. subtilis* for ethylene oxide sterilizers.
- If the test is positive for growth, immediately rechallenge the sterilizer.
- If there is a subsequent abnormal result of biologic indicators, take the sterilizer out of service until the problem is corrected and a normal reading is obtained.
- Recall and reprocess suspected load items if a sterilizer malfunction in found (AORN, 1992, *III*:20–2—20–3).

Test Packs for Biologic Challenge of Steam Sterilization Monitoring

- A routine test pack consists of three muslin gowns, 12 towels, 30 4 × 4 inch gauze sponges, five laparotomy sponges, and one muslin drape sheet.
- Place two biologic indicators in the center of the pack.
- Place a chemical indicator one towel above or below the biologic indicators.
- Place the test pack on edge at the front bottom, near the door, in a routinely loaded gravity displacement sterilizer.

- Place the test pack on edge at the front bottom, near the door, by itself in a prevacuum steam sterilizer (AORN, 1992, *III*:20–3).

Biologic Challenge Test for Ethylene Oxide Sterilizers

- A general-purpose ethylene oxide sterilizer is a chamber-type sterilizer that provides humidity adjustment during the sterilization cycle.
- Make a general test pack of four clean surgical towels, each folded in thirds and then halved to create six layers per towel.
- Place these on top of one another.
- Add one adult plastic airway, a 10-inch section of latex tubing with an internal diameter of 3/16 inch, and two plastic or glass syringes with biologic indicators placed in the barrels to the center of the towels.
- Insert the plungers into the barrels of the syringes. The plunger diaphragm should not touch the biologic indicator.
- Sequentially wrap the pack with two 24 x 24 inch wrappers and secure with tape.
- Chemical indicators and a biologic indicator may be used in the same sterilization cycle as the general test pack (AORN, 1992, *III*:20–3).

SPECIAL PURPOSE
- A special-purpose ethylene oxide sterilization system requires prehumidification of items to be sterilized and usually operates at atmospheric pressure.
- Special test packs include one 10-inch length of latex tubing $\frac{3}{16}$ inch in diameter and two syringes with biologic indicators enclosed in the syringe barrel and the syringe tip open.
- Wrap in single-thickness wrapper and close with tape.

Challenge Test Pack

- Use a challenge test pack placed in an 80 to 100 cubic foot chamber.
- Five test packs are used. Place one in the center front and the others in diagonally opposite corners in the upper and lower levels.
- For a 40 to 79 cubic foot chamber, use three test packs. Place one each in the center, front section, and rear upper section.
- For a 16 to 39 cubic foot chamber, use two test packs. Place one in the rear corner and one in the front corner.
- For a chamber of less than 16 cubic feet, place one pack in the front of the chamber near the door.

Routine Test Pack

- In a routine test pack, place one biologic indicator in a plastic syringe of sufficient size that the indicator does not touch the

plunger. This syringe has an open tip and is placed inside a folded, clean, 100% cotton towel.
- Put these articles into a single-peel pouch wrapper and place in the center of the load.
- After the sterilization cycle, remove biologic test pack indicators and controls and incubate according to the manufacturer's recommendations (AORN, 1992, *III*:20–3).

Sterilizer Performance Records

- Label each package to be sterilized with a lot control number, which designates the sterilizer used, the date of sterilization, the cycle number, and an expiration date.
- Keep sterilizer performance records for each sterilizer.
- These should include the contents of each load as to general category, duration and temperature of the sterilization phase, identification of the operator, results of biologic testing, a time and temperature recording chart for the sterilizer, and a record of repairs and preventive maintenance (AORN, 1992, *III*:20–6).

Preventive Maintenance

- Preventive maintenance procedures are outlined by the manufacturer of the sterilizer. In general, areas that need attention are air filters, steam traps, drain pipes, and door gaskets.

Daily Inspection and Cleaning

- Daily care of sterilizer is done while sterilizer is cool.
- Remove the chamber drain strainer and eliminate debris and sediment.
- Wash and rinse all internal surfaces of the sterilizer, using only the recommended cleaning agent.
- Clean door gaskets.
- Observe for evidence of gasket failure leaks, blowing of steam, water on the interior of the autoclave, and low pressures.
- Check for proper functioning of the recording chart and pen.

Weekly and Routine Inspection and Cleaning

- Weekly inspection and cleaning should include discharge system and accessories.
- Routine maintenance is done at least every 6 months. This includes inspection, servicing, and calibration (AORN, 1992, *III*:20–6).

Documenting Procedures

- Keep permanent records regarding the results of biologic monitoring, autoclave graphs and recording charts, load contents, and load control numbers.

- Keep maintenance records for each sterilizer. Include
  1. Date of service
  2. Model and serial number
  3. A description of the service performed
  4. The name of the individual performing the service
  5. A description and quantity of the parts replaced
  6. The results of biologic indicator and/or a Bowie-Dick test after the repair
  7. The name of the authorized person requesting service
  8. The signature of the person acknowledging completed work
- Label each item or pack intended for use as a sterile product with
  1. A lot control number, which designates the sterilizer identification number
  2. The date of sterilization
  3. The cycle number
- Ensure that policies and procedures are available to address procedures for checking items that may be outdated, damaged, or contaminated (AORN, 1992, *III*:20–5).

POSITIONING THE PATIENT

The perioperative nurse demonstrates competency to position by placing the patient in the
- Supine position
- Trendelenburg position
- Reverse Trendelenburg position
- Low lithotomy position
- High lithotomy position
- Lateral decubitus position
- Prone position
- Jackknife position
- Sitting position

Considerations for All Surgical Positions
Communication
- Communication with the patient and members of the operative team is essential.
- Inform the patient of the positioning procedure during the patient teaching session.
- Specific intraoperative patient requirements should be communicated with other members of the operative team (AORN, 1992, *III*:14–1).

Prepare the Operating Room Bed
- Before transferring the patient, if necessary, modify the OR bed.

- Ensure that the OR bed is functioning properly, clean, free from hazards, and padded (AORN, 1992, *III*:14–1).
- Check that pads are of equal height.
- Lock the OR bed in place.
- Collect all required positioning devices and attachments. Check that devices and attachments are functional, clean, and free from hazards.
- Attach a padded table extension if the patient's body will extend beyond the end of the OR bed.
- Transfer the patient to the OR bed.

Center the Patient on the OR Bed

- Align the patient's head, spine, and legs. Ensure that the patient's legs are not crossed.
- Apply the safety strap at least 2 inches above the knees without excessive pressure.
- Insert a hand between the strap and the thighs to check for excessive pressure.

Place the Patient's Arms on the Arm Boards

- Attach the arm boards to the OR bed at less than a 90-degree angle to the body.
- Secure each arm with a safety strap.
- If the palms are placed at the sides, turn them toward the patient's sides with the fingers extended.
- Pad the arms and tuck them with the drawsheet.
- Check the elbows to ensure that they are not flexed or resting on the metal edge of the OR bed.
- Ensure that the fingers are clear of the OR bed breaks and other possible hazards.
- Pad bony prominences.

Moving the Anesthetized Patient

- Check with the anesthetist before positioning or repositioning the anesthetized patient.
- Do not move the patient unless adequate assistance is available.
- Move the patient slowly, as a coordinated team.
- Reassess the patient for body alignment and tissue integrity (AORN, 1992, *III*:14–3) before draping.
- Examine the safety strap to ensure that it is secure and not constrictive.

Supine Position (Figs. 31 and 32)
Supplies and Equipment
PRIMARY
- Arm boards

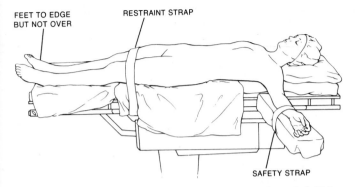

FEET TO EDGE
BUT NOT OVER

RESTRAINT STRAP

SAFETY STRAP

FIGURE 31 Supine position with arms extended. (From Fuller, J. R. [1986]. *Surgical technology: Principles and practice* [2nd ed]. Philadelphia: W. B. Saunders.)

- Arm restraints
- Pillow or headrest
- Padding for bony prominences (foam, sheepskin, blankets, pillows)
- Safety strap
SUPPLEMENTARY
- Padded footboard
- Pelvic wedge
- OR bed extension
- Toboggans

Procedure

- After the transfer, align the patient's head, neck, spine, and legs.
- Ensure that the legs are not crossed and are slightly apart.
- Secure the safety belt above the knees.
- Check that the patient is not resting on any unpadded surfaces.

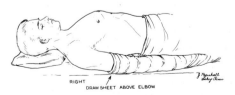

RIGHT
DRAW SHEET ABOVE ELBOW

FIGURE 32 Supine position with arms tucked. (From Ginsberg, F. [1966]. *A manual of operating room technology.* Philadelphia: J. B. Lippincott.)

- Check that extremities are secured away from the OR bed joints (breaks) and attachments.
- When using arm boards, do not abduct the patient's arms more than 90 degrees.
- Secure the arms to the arm boards with safety straps.
- If the arms are to be placed at the patient's sides, turn the palms toward the body or the bed and secure the full length of the arms with a drawsheet or a padded toboggan (McAlpine and Sechel, 1987, pp. 317, 319).
- Apply protective padding to all areas that are susceptible to injury.
- Place a small pad under the patient's head, lower lumbar area, and heels and avoid hyperextending the knees (Smith, 1987, p. 34).
- For pregnant or obese patients, place a small pelvic wedge under the right side of the patient to relieve pressure on the vena cava (Smith, 1987, p. 35).
- If needed, attach a padded footboard to the bed.

Trendelenburg Position (Fig. 33)
Supplies and Equipment
- See Supine Position

Procedure
- Position the patient as described for the supine position.
- If the knee section of the OR bed is to be lowered to minimize pressure on the calves and knee joints, position the top edge of

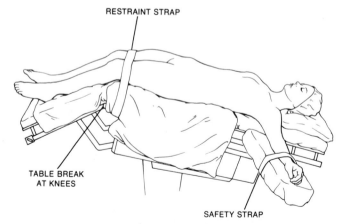

FIGURE 33 Trendelenburg position. (From Fuller, J. R. [1986]. *Surgical technology: Principles and practice* [2nd ed]. Philadelphia: W. B. Saunders.)

the patient's knees below the hinge, at a distance approximately equal to the thickness of the OR bed pad and x-ray tunnel (Prentice and Martin, 1987, pp. 130–131; Rothrock, 1987, p. 266).
- Tilt the bed, feet up and head down, to the desired angle.

Reverse Trendelenburg Position (Fig. 34)
Supplies and Equipment
- See Supine Position

Procedure
- Position the patient as described for the supine position.
- Attach a padded footboard to keep the patient from sliding toward the foot of the OR bed.
- Tilt the bed, feet down and head up, to the desired angle.

High Lithotomy Position (Fig. 35)
Personnel Requirements
Two persons are required to position the patient in the high lithotomy position.

Supplies and Equipment
- See Supine Position
- Protective leg coverings (foam boots, towels)
- Stirrups
- Stirrup holders
- Rail sockets

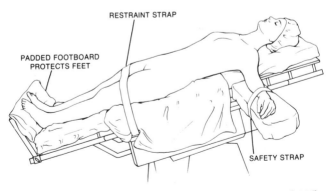

FIGURE 34 Reverse Trendelenburg position. (From Fuller, J. R. [1986]. *Surgical technology: Principles and practice* [2nd ed]. Philadelphia: W. B. Saunders.)

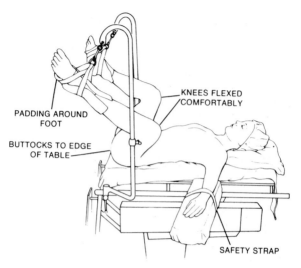

Figure 35   High lithotomy position. (From Fuller, J. R. [1986]. *Surgical technology: Principles and practice* [2nd ed]. Philadelphia: W. B. Saunders.)

Procedure

ADJUST THE OPERATING ROOM BED AND TRANSFER THE PATIENT
- Before transferring the patient, adjust the OR bed.
- Release the head section of the mattress pad and pull the head-piece and mattress pad out.
- Attach the headpiece and mattress to the foot of the OR bed.
- Refit the bedsheet to the OR bed.
- Transfer and prepare the patient for administration of anesthesia in the supine position as described for interventions for all surgical positions.
- Apply protective padding to the patient's feet and lower legs.
- Use other protective padding as described for interventions for all surgical positions.

ATTACH THE STIRRUPS
- Attach the stirrup holders to the OR bed above the knee break hinge.
- Insert the stirrups into the holders and tighten.
- Adjust the stirrups to the appropriate height; ensure that they are level and secure.

PLACE THE PATIENT IN THE HIGH LITHOTOMY POSITION
- After the patient is anesthetized, remove the safety strap from the legs.

- Grasp the sole of one foot in one hand, supporting the leg at the knee with the other hand.
- Instruct the assistant to perform the same maneuver for the other leg.
- Together with the assistant, *slowly* flex the legs toward the abdomen, then slightly externally rotate the hips and secure the feet to the stirrups (Fuller, 1986, p. 73).
- Cover the patient's genitalia and perineum with a towel or sheet.

COMPLETE MODIFICATION OF THE OPERATING ROOM BED

- Remove the headrest and the leg section of the OR bed.
- Place the headrest and the leg section on a clean surface outside the surgeon's work area.
- Check that the patient's fingers are not in the hinges of the bed.
- Lower the leg section of the OR bed.

Repositioning the Patient Before Surgery

- Remove the arm board straps and fold the patient's arms across the abdomen.
- Have the assistant stand by the patient to protect the arms.
- Stand between the patient's legs and move the patient to the edge of the OR bed break by placing the hands and arms under the patient's buttocks and gently lifting using proper body mechanics, or with another team member lift the patient with the drawsheet.
- Move the arm boards and resecure the patient's arms.

Repositioning the Patient After Surgery

- Check to ensure that the patient's hands and fingers are not extending beyond the OR bed break.
- Elevate the leg section to the horizontal position.
- Replace the mattress pad on the leg section.
- Put the head section and mattress pad back on the foot of the bed.
- Have the assistant stand on the opposite side of the OR bed and perform the same maneuvers for the other leg.
- When given clearance by the anesthetist, grasp the patient's legs and remove the stirrup strap.
- With one hand under the patient's heel and the other under the knee, *slowly* extend the legs and lower them together.
- Reapply the safety strap securely across the thighs.
- Cover the patient with a warm sheet or blanket.
- Remove the positioning equipment from the OR bed.

Low Lithotomy Position (Fig. 36)
Staffing Requirements

The perioperative nurse and an assistant are the minimal nursing staff needed to position the patient.

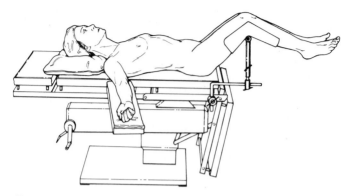

Figure 36 Low lithotomy position. (Modified from Martin, J. T. [Ed.] [1987]. *Positioning in anesthesia and surgery* [2nd ed]. Philadelphia: W. B. Saunders.)

Supplies and Equipment

- See supplies and equipment for the high lithotomy position.

Procedure

ADJUST THE OPERATING ROOM BED AND TRANSFER THE PATIENT

- Adjust the OR bed as described for the high lithotomy position.
- Transfer and prepare the patient for administration of anesthesia in the supine position as described under interventions for all surgical positions.

APPLY PROTECTIVE DEVICES

- Apply protective padding to the patient's feet and lower legs.
- Apply additional protective padding as described under interventions for all surgical positions.

ATTACH THE LEG HOLDERS

- Attach the rail socket to the OR bed above the knee break hinge. Insert the leg holders into the rail socket and tighten. Adjust the leg holders to the appropriate height; ensure that they are level and secure.

PLACE THE PATIENT IN THE LOW LITHOTOMY POSITION

- After the patient is anesthetized, remove the safety strap from the legs.
- Grasp the sole of one foot in one hand, supporting the leg at the knee with the other hand.
- Instruct the assistant to perform the same maneuver with the other leg. Together with the assistant, *slowly* flex the legs toward the abdomen, then slightly externally rotate the hips and secure the legs to the leg holders (Fuller, 1986, p. 73; Kropp, 1987, p. 54).

- Ensure that the thighs are at an obtuse angle to the trunk.
- Cover the patient's genitalia and perineum with a towel or a sheet.
- Complete modification of the OR bed as described for the high lithotomy position.
- Reposition the patient if necessary as described for the high lithotomy position.

Repositioning After Surgery
- Check to ensure that the patient's hands and fingers are not extending beyond the OR bed break.
- Elevate the leg section to the horizontal position.
- Replace the mattress pad on the leg section and put the head section and mattress pad back on the foot of the bed.
- Have the assistant stand on the opposite side of the OR bed and perform the same maneuvers for the other leg.
- When given clearance by the anesthetist, place one hand under the patient's heel and the other under the knee, *slowly* lift the legs off the leg holder, extend the legs, and lower them together.
- Reapply the safety strap.
- Cover the patient with a warm sheet or blanket.
- Remove the positioning equipment from the OR bed.

Lateral Decubitus Position (Fig. 37)
Staffing Requirements
The perioperative nurse and three assistants are the minimum nursing staff needed to position the patient.

Supplies and Equipment
- Pillows
- Headrest
- Padding for bony prominences (foam, sheepskin, blankets, pillows)
- Arm boards
- A safety strap
- Beanbag

Procedure
TRANSFER THE PATIENT TO THE OPERATING ROOM BED
- Transfer and prepare the patient for administration of anesthesia in the supine position as described for interventions for all surgical positions.

PREPARE THE ASSISTANTS
- Ensure that the assistants understand their individual roles.
- The circulating nurse and one assistant stand on the right side of the OR bed if the patient's left side will be facing down. If the

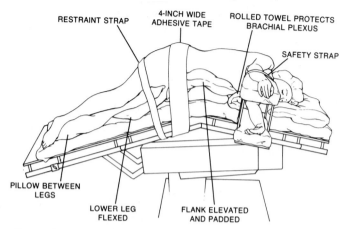

RESTRAINT STRAP
4-INCH WIDE ADHESIVE TAPE
ROLLED TOWEL PROTECTS BRACHIAL PLEXUS
SAFETY STRAP
PILLOW BETWEEN LEGS
LOWER LEG FLEXED
FLANK ELEVATED AND PADDED

FIGURE 37 Lateral position. (From Fuller, J. R. [1986]. *Surgical technology: Principles and practice* [2nd ed]. Philadelphia: W. B. Saunders.)

patient's right side will be facing down, the circulating nurse and assistant stand on the left side of the OR bed. The other two assistants stand on the opposite side of the OR bed, one across from the circulating nurse and the other near the foot of the OR bed.

TURN AND POSITION THE PATIENT

- The anesthetist controls the head and neck and initiates the movement.
- After the patient's arms are placed at his or her sides, the circulating nurse and assistant reach under the patient's shoulders and hips, lift slightly, and draw the patient's far shoulder and hip toward the middle of the OR bed. Next they concurrently rotate the patient to the lateral position.
- The assistant across from the circulating nurse helps rotate the patient. The assistant near the foot of the OR bed controls the patient's legs.
- Support the patient until after the anesthetist has reestablished ventilation. Place a rolled towel or other type of padding (axillary roll) under the patient below the axilla, not in the axilla (Thomas, 1987, p. 151).
- Secure the patient with tape, beanbags, rolls, or other type of support. Flex the downside leg at the knee to add stability.
- Place a pillow or padding between the patient's legs. After positioning the patient, ensure that the patient's head, neck, and spine are in proper alignment and that the axillary roll is in the

proper position below the axilla, the genitalia and breast are free from pressure, the legs and knees are padded, no part of the patient's anatomy is resting on an unpadded surface, and the extremities are secured away from the OR bed joints (breaks) and attachments.
- Stabilize and secure the patient's body to the OR bed.

Prone Position (Fig. 38)

- Typically, the patient is placed under general anesthesia on the gurney before being transferred to the OR bed. However, the patient may be anesthetized on the OR bed and then rotated into the prone position.

Staffing Requirements

- The perioperative nurse and three assistants are the minimal nursing staff needed to position the patient.

Supplies and Equipment

- Pillows
- Headrest
- Chest rolls or a supporting frame (Relton, Wilson, and so on)
- Padding for bony prominences and the dorsa of the feet (foam, sheepskin, blankets, pillows), arm boards
- Arm restraints
- Safety strap
- Face rest (horseshoe, Mayfield, and so on)
- Padded knee rest
- Table extension

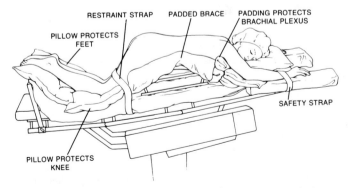

FIGURE 38   Prone position. (From Fuller, J. R. [1986]. *Surgical technology: Principles and practice* [2nd ed]. Philadelphia: W. B. Saunders.)

Procedure

TRANSFER THE PATIENT TO THE OPERATING ROOM BED

- Transfer and prepare the patient for anesthesia administration in the supine position as described for interventions for all surgical positions.

TURN THE PATIENT ON THE OPERATING ROOM BED

- Prepare the assistants by ensuring that they understand their individual roles. The circulating nurse and one assistant stand on one side of the OR bed and the other two assistants stand on the opposite side of the OR bed.
- The anesthetist controls the head and neck and initiates the movement. After the patient's arms are placed at his or her sides, the circulating nurse and assistant reach under the patient's shoulders and hips, lift slightly, and draw the patient's far shoulder and hip toward the middle of the OR bed.
- The nurse and assistant concurrently rotate the patient to the lateral position. The assistant across from the circulating nurse helps rotate the patient. The assistant near the foot of the bed should control the legs. Continue rotating the patient while centering the trunk on the OR bed.
- Support the patient until after the anesthetist has reestablished ventilation. Place the positioning devices under the patient (Martin, 1987, p. 199).

PLACE THE PATIENT IN POSITION

- After turning the patient, ensure that the chest rolls extend from the acromioclavicular joint to the iliac crest and do not impinge on the chest expansion (Gruendemann, 1987, p. 62).
- Ensure that the breasts are displaced medially on the chest rolls (Martin, 1987, pp. 216–217).
- Check that the head, neck, spine, and legs are in proper alignment.
- Ensure that the legs are uncrossed and slightly apart.
- Check and free genitalia from pressure.
- Pad iliac crests and knees.
- Support the dorsum of the foot with a pillow to prevent pressure on the toes.
- Ensure that no part of the patient's anatomy is resting on an unpadded surface. Ensure that the extremities are secured away from the OR bed joints (breaks) and attachments. Secure the body to the bed.

POSITION THE ARMS

- If arm boards are used, the patient's arms "should be rotated cephalad in a plane roughly parallel to the sagittal plane of the body" (Martin, 1987, p. 202).
- The arms are positioned above the patient's head with the elbows flexed and secured to the arm boards.

- If the arms are placed at the patient's side, the palms should be turned toward the body or the bed, and the full length of the arms needs to be secured by a drawsheet or a padded toboggan.

REASSESS THE PATIENT
- Reassess the patient before draping.
- Ensure that the chest rolls extend from the clavicle to the iliac crest and do not impinge on the chest expansion.
- Check that the female breasts are displaced medially on the chest rolls.
- The body should be properly aligned and the safety strap in place.
- The arms should be properly secured and placed on the arm boards or at the patient's side.
- Check that there is no pressure on the genitalia.
- The dorsum of the foot should be supported to prevent pressure on the toes.

Jackknife (Kraske) Position (Fig. 39)
Staffing Requirements
- The perioperative nurse and three assistants are the minimal nursing staff needed to position the patient.

Supplies and Equipment
- Pillows
- Headrest
- Chest rolls or a supporting frame (Relton, Wilson, and so on)
- Padding for bony prominences and the dorsa of the feet (foam, sheepskin, blankets, pillows)
- Arm boards

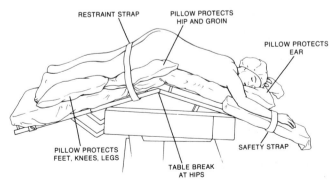

RESTRAINT STRAP

PILLOW PROTECTS HIP AND GROIN

PILLOW PROTECTS EAR

PILLOW PROTECTS FEET, KNEES, LEGS

TABLE BREAK AT HIPS

SAFETY STRAP

FIGURE 39 Jackknife (Kraske) position. (From Fuller, J. R. [1986]. *Surgical technology: Principles and practice* [2nd ed]. Philadelphia: W. B. Saunders.)

- Arm restraints
- Safety strap
- Face rest (horseshoe, Mayfield, and so on)
- Padded knee rest
- Table extension

Procedure

TRANSFER THE PATIENT TO THE OPERATING ROOM BED
- Transfer and prepare the patient for administration of anesthesia in the supine position as described for interventions for all surgical positions.

TURN AND POSITION THE PATIENT
- Ensure that the assistants understand their individual roles.
- The circulating nurse and one assistant stand on one side of the OR bed and the other two assistants stand on the opposite side of the OR bed.
- Position the patient as described for the prone position.

ADJUST THE OPERATING ROOM BED
- Ensure that the patient's hips are positioned over the OR bed break.
- Check that there is no pressure on the patient's genitalia.
- Reverse flex the OR bed until the patient is in an inverted V position.

REASSESS THE PATIENT
- Reassess the patient before draping for any potential discrepancies as described for the prone position.

Sitting Position (Fig. 40)
Staffing Requirements
- The perioperative nurse is the minimal staff needed.
- Additional staffing requirements need to be noted on the perioperative nursing care plan.

Supplies and Equipment
- Arm boards
- Arm restraints
- Head holder (e.g., skull clamp, Mayfield, Gardner, with sterile skull pins)
- Padding for bony prominences (foam, sheepskin, blankets, pillows)
- Padded footboard
- Safety strap
- Antigravity suit
- Medical antishock trousers
- Elastic bandages

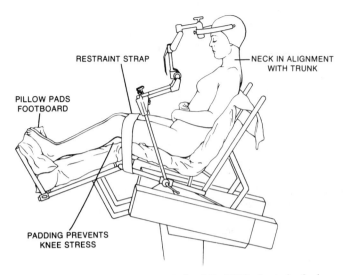

FIGURE 40 Sitting position. (From Fuller, J. R. [1986]. *Surgical technology: Principles and practice* [2nd ed]. Philadelphia: W. B. Saunders.)

- Table extension
- Toboggans

Procedure

TRANSFER THE PATIENT TO THE OPERATING ROOM BED

- Transfer and prepare the patient for administration of anesthesia in the supine position as described for interventions for all surgical positions.

PREPARE THE PATIENT

- Before placing the patient in the sitting position, wrap both legs of the patient to the groin with elastic bandages or compression stockings.
- The surgeon may request that an antigravity suit or medical antishock trousers be applied.
- Generously pad the patient under the buttocks and place padding under each heel.
- A padded footboard should be attached to the end of the OR bed (Rothrock, 1987, p. 290).

MODIFY THE OPERATING ROOM BED TO THE SITTING POSITION

- Elevate the patient's back, flex the bed, and lower the footpiece.
- After the patient is in position, place the patient's arms on a pillow that has been set on her or his lap and secure with 3-inch ad-

hesive tape attached to the OR bed frame. Pad each elbow with rubber.
- If available, place the patient's arms in arm holders.
- Attach the accessories for the skull clamp (Rothrock, 1987, p. 290).

REASSESS THE PATIENT
- Check the patient for alignment.
- If the patient is male, check to ensure that the scrotum and penis are not twisted or compressed between the legs (Rothrock, 1987, p. 290).

Documentation and Communication Procedures

- Include a preoperative nursing history, assessment, and care plan. At a minimum, the assessment should include the following:
  1. Physical limitations
  2. Weight
  3. Height
  4. Nutritional status
  5. Skin condition
  6. Preexisting disease
  7. Type and length of procedure (AORN, 1992, *III*:14–7)
- The nurses' notes should contain information about the interventions used to eliminate, diminish, or alter the patient risk factors identified in the care plan. The intraoperative nursing record should include the following:
  1. Position
  2. Safety and security measures
  3. The use and the location of positioning devices (AORN, 1992, *III*:14–3)
- Postoperatively, assess and document the patient's physical condition.

HANDLING CULTURES AND SPECIMENS

The perioperative nurse demonstrates competency to handle cultures and specimens by correctly
- Providing supplies and equipment needed for the collection of cultures and specimens
- Labeling culture and tissue specimen containers
- Completing laboratory slips
- Documenting the collection of cultures and specimens on the patient's operative record
- Establishing chain of custody for cultures and tissue specimens
- Obtaining and processing cultures for examination
- Storing, preserving, and maintaining tissue

- Directing the transfer of cultures and specimens to the laboratory
- Communicating intraoperative pathology reports to the surgeon

Considerations

- Consider all cultures and specimens as potentially infectious (Table 19).
- Wear gloves at all times when handling cultures and specimens.
- After removing gloves, wash hands.
- Avoid contaminating the exterior surface of culture tubes or specimen containers with blood or other body fluids.
- If contamination occurs, disinfect exterior surfaces of tubes or containers with a tuberculocidal hospital-grade disinfectant or a 1:10 dilution of household bleach before they are removed from the operating room (AORN, 1992, *III*:17–2).
- If tubes or containers cannot be disinfected, place them in an impervious clear bag for transportation to the laboratory and note on the label that the exterior surface of the tube or container is contaminated.

TABLE **19**
Common Pathogens of Nosocomial Infections

Aerobic bacteria	Microaerophilic bacteria
Gram-positive cocci	Gram-positive cocci
Staphylococcus aureus	Hemolytic streptococci
S. epidermidis	Nonhemolytic streptococci
Streptococcus group B	Anaerobic bacteria
Streptococcus group D	Gram-positive cocci
Gram-negative cocci	*Peptostreptococcus*
Neisseria gonorrhoeae	*Peptococcus*
Gram-positive bacilli	Gram-positive bacilli
Bacillus subtilis	*Clostridium tetani*
Mycobacterium tuberculosis	*C. welchii*
Gram-negative bacilli	Gram-negative bacilli
Escherichia coli	*Bacteroides* species
Klebsiella pneumoniae	*B. fragilis*
Pseudomonas aeruginosa	Nonbacterial microorganisms
P. cepacia	Viruses
Proteus vulgaris	Herpesvirus
Serratia marcescens	Hepatitis virus
Salmonella species	Human immunodeficiency virus
Alcaligenes faecalis	Fungi
Haemophilus influenzae	*Candida albicans*
Enterobacter species	*Histoplasma capsulatum*
	Phycomycosis species

Adapted from Atkinson, L. J., Kohn, M. L. (1986). *Berry and Kohn's introduction to operating room technique* (6th ed) (p. 103). New York: McGraw-Hill. With permission of Mosby–Year Book.

- Prevent contamination of documents such as labels and laboratory slips (AORN, 1992, *III*:1–2). If they become contaminated, prepare fresh documents.

Supplies and Equipment
- Addressograph
- Labels and laboratory slips (histology, cytology, aerobic, anaerobic, and acid-fast)
- Culture tubes (aerobic and anaerobic)
- Test tubes with caps
- Blood culture bottles
- Petri dishes
- Tissue specimen containers
- Formalin

Providing Supplies and Equipment
- Gather supplies and equipment needed for cultures and specimens before the patient is transferred to the OR bed.
- Determine the types of supplies and equipment needed by assessing the patient, reviewing the patient's record, checking the surgeon's preference card, and questioning the surgeon concerning specific culture and specimen needs.
- If appropriate, contact laboratory personnel or pathologists to make arrangements for special tests or procedures.

Labeling Culture and Specimen Containers
- The label should contain at least the following information:
    1. Patient's name
    2. Patient's identification number
    3. Physician's name
    4. Source of the culture or type of tissue specimen
    5. Date and time of collection

Completing Laboratory Slips
The following information should be recorded on the laboratory slip:
- Patient's name
- Patient's identification number
- Physician's name
- Culture or tissue source (specific)
- Date and time of collection
- Patient's medical diagnosis
- Patient's unit room number
- Identification of the study requested

- Other pertinent information such as antibiotics being administered

Documenting the Collection of Cultures and Specimens

The operative record should reflect the source of the culture or the type of specimen, the time of collection, and the studies requested.

- Note the final disposition of the culture and specimen.
- If a specimen is not obtained, this also should be reflected on the operative record.
- Although not part of the operative record, laboratory slips, if returned to the OR during the intraoperative period with study results, should be placed in the patient's chart.

Establishing Chain of Custody

The following information should be recorded in the log book:

- Patient's name
- Patient's identification number
- Physician's name
- Source of culture or type of tissue specimen or object
- Person logging the specimen
- Date and time of log in
- Person receiving the specimen
- Date and time of disposition

Collecting and Preparing Cultures for Examination
General Guidelines

- When obtaining fluid, tissue, or other material for culture, obtain enough specimen to permit performance of all tests requested by the physician.
- Use sterile equipment and receptacles so as not to contaminate the specimen with exogenous microorganisms.
- Maintain integrity of the culture specimen.
- Do not allow the specimen contact with chemicals, germicides, or disinfectants that may compromise laboratory processing and invalidate study results.
- If multiple studies are ordered, obtain one culture for each test (Santa Rosa Hospital, 1988, #161, p. 0003).

Aerobic Cultures

- Use a sterile culture tube with a cotton swab to obtain an aerobic culture during the operative procedure.
- After the surgeon notifies the nursing team that she or he wants aerobic cultures taken, prepare (circulator) the culture system. Two methods of obtaining the culture are acceptable.

First method

- The circulator removes the sterile tube from the package.
- The bottom of the tube is held with one hand, while the other hand carefully removes the top of the tube and exposes the distal end of the cotton swab.
- The scrub person grasps the end of the swab attached to the top and pulls it from the culture tube while avoiding touching or contaminating the cotton swabs.
- If the culture is to be taken immediately, the circulating nurse stands adjacent to the sterile field, tube and cap in hand, ready to accept the swab.
- If the culture will be taken later, the circulating nurse recaps the tube.
- After the culture is taken, the scrub person carefully inserts the swab into the tube, which is held by the circulating nurse.
- The circulating nurse then recaps the tube and crushes the media ampule at the midpoint of the bottom tube by gently squeezing the tube over the ampule.
- Next, the circulating nurse pushes on the cap to ensure that the swab tip contacts the moistened pledgets.
- The tube is labeled and sent to the laboratory with the appropriate laboratory slip.
- If done correctly, this method is preferable because it ensures that the exterior of the culture tube is not contaminated.

Second Method

- The circulating nurse aseptically delivers the culture tube and swab to the sterile field.
- The scrub person removes the cotton swab and passes it to the surgeon.
- After the culture is taken, the surgeon or the scrub person inserts the swab into the tube.
- The scrub person recaps the tube and passes it off the sterile field to the circulating nurse.
- Wearing gloves, the circulating nurse receives the tube, decontaminates it with a tuberculocidal hospital-grade disinfectant or a 1:10 dilution of household bleach, breaks the media ampule, pushes the swab into the media, attaches a label, and sends the tube to the laboratory with the appropriate laboratory slip.

Anaerobic Cultures

- Obtain anaerobic cultures in such a manner that the specimen is not in contact with air for a long period of time.
- If a swab is used to obtain the specimen, use care to ensure that it is not aerated.

- Send fluid for anaerobic cultures to the laboratory in an anaerobic culture transport system or a syringe with all air removed.
- Use a sterile plastic tube for tissue obtained for anaerobic study. In such cases, however, immediately send the specimen to the laboratory. Delay in dispatching the specimen can hinder the culturing process (Santa Rosa Hospital, 1988, #166, p. 0002).
- The circulating nurse aseptically delivers the anaerobic culture system to the sterile field.
- The scrub person pulls the cap with the swab attached out of the tube and passes it to the surgeon.
- After obtaining the culture, the surgeon or the scrub person inserts the swab into the tube.
- While recapping the tube, the scrub person pushes the cap firmly onto the tube with a downward motion.
- The gloved circulating nurse receives the anaerobic culture tube from the sterile field, decontaminates it as described for aerobic culture tubes, attaches a label, and immediately sends it to the laboratory with the appropriate laboratory slip.

Using a Syringe to Collect Fluid

- When the surgeon asks for a syringe to collect fluid for an anaerobic or aerobic culture, the circulating nurse aseptically delivers an appropriate-sized syringe to the sterile field. If a needle is needed for collection, a large-gauge needle should be used.
- If the surgeon aspirates the fluid without a needle, the scrub person recaps the syringe and passes it to the gloved circulating nurse. Preferably, the scrub person drops the syringe into an impervious container, such as a plastic bag, held by the circulating nurse.
- Once the syringe is passed off the field, avoid decontaminating the syringe because ejection or leakage of syringe contents is possible by inadvertent pushing or pulling of the plunger by the circulating nurse.
- The circulating nurse labels the container with patient and specimen data, marks it to alert laboratory personnel that the syringe is contaminated, and sends the container to the laboratory with the appropriate laboratory slip.

Gram Stains

- Use an aerobic culture tube to collect cultures for Gram stains.
- Immediately send cultures for Gram stains to the laboratory for smear and fixation.
- An appropriate laboratory slip is forwarded with the culture.

Spinal Fluid

- Fluid removed during a spinal tap may be sent to the laboratory in sterile tubes.
- Ensure that sufficient fluid is collected for the requested study.
- Guidelines for minimal amounts include
  1. Aerobic culture and smear: 1.5 to 2 ml
  2. Fungus culture: 1 ml
  3. Acid-fast culture and smear: 2 ml
- If cell count, cell differentiation, glucose, or protein studies are requested, separate tubes must be sent.
- Label the tubes and send with the appropriate laboratory requisition slips immediately to the laboratory.

Acid-fast Cultures and Smears

- Acid-fast cultures and smears are sent in the aerobic transport system.
- One swab is needed for each test. The specimen is labeled and sent immediately to the laboratory with the proper laboratory requisition slip (Santa Rosa Hospital, 1988, #171, p. 0002).

Fungus Cultures

- Collect fluid or pus in a syringe.
- Use of a dry, sterile Petri dish is also acceptable.
- Collect as much of the specimen as possible.
- Like other specimens, the specimen for mycologic studies is labeled and immediately sent to the laboratory with the appropriate laboratory slip.

Collecting and Preparing Tissue for Examination
General Guidelines

- Handle all specimens carefully and as little as possible.
- Do not shake fluid specimens.
- Do not crush or tear specimens.
- When transferring a specimen with an instrument, protect the specimen from tearing or damage (Atkinson and Kohn, 1986, p. 174).
- Keep tissue in a near-natural state, particularly tissues sent for frozen section examination.
- Prevent specimen drying.
- The scrub person places the specimen in a container, such as an emesis basin.
- While the specimen is on the sterile field, the scrub person keeps the specimen damp by frequently wetting it with normal saline solution.

Permanent Specimens

- All tissue or other objects removed from the patient are sent to the laboratory as permanent specimens.
- Exceptions to this guideline are dictated by hospital policy.
- After removal, hand specimens off the sterile field as soon as possible. This helps prevent inadvertent discarding of the specimen during cleanup after the end of the procedure.
- After receiving permission from the surgeon, the scrub person passes the specimen to the gloved circulating nurse.
- For transfer of the specimen to an appropriate-sized container, the emesis basin is tipped, thus causing the specimen to slide from the basin into the container.
- If necessary, use an instrument to transfer the specimen to the container.
- Avoid splashing if the container is already filled with formalin.
- When pouring formalin over the specimen, exercise care to avoid splashing.
- Completely cover the specimen with formalin. Exceptions are bladder stones or gallstones. These are sent dry to prevent decomposition.
- When the size of a specimen makes it difficult to see, the scrub nurse places the specimen on a piece of material that provides contrast.
- Telfa is suitable and may be submerged in formalin and sent to the laboratory.
- Each container should contain only one specimen.
- If specimens are bilateral, such as fallopian tubes, label each specimen as left or right. Also make medial and lateral designations.
- Place specimens that are too large for standard containers in an appropriate-sized basin and transport immediately to the laboratory with the appropriate paperwork.
- Avoid contamination of the transporter and laboratory personnel by placing the basin containing the specimen in a clear impervious bag.
- Ensure that all permanent specimens are appropriately labeled.
- Attach the laboratory slip to the container with a rubber band or place it in a readily accessible place near the specimen container.

Specimens for Frozen Section

- When a frozen section examination is anticipated, notify the pathologist before the surgical procedure begins.
- After the specimen is obtained from the patient, the scrub person passes it off the sterile field on a section of dampened Telfa, on a towel, or in a container such as an emesis basin.

- Do not pass specimens off the field on a counted sponge.
- The gloved circulating nurse receives the specimen and transfers it to an appropriate-sized dry container.
- Do not place the specimen in fluid such as formalin or saline solution.
- Attach a label to the container and immediately take the specimen to the pathology department.

Storing, Preserving, and Maintaining Tissue

- Assess potential donors to ensure that they are free from transmissible infection, malignant disease, autoimmune disease, neurologic disease of unknown cause, and human-derived growth hormone.
- Policies regarding banking of donor and recipient tissue vary from hospital to hospital.
- Remove tissue under strict aseptic conditions and store in a controlled environment.

Acceptable methods (AORN, 1992, *III*:21–3)

- For short-term storage, "place skin in an isotonic solution (e.g., normal saline or balanced salt solution) or tissue medium and refrigerate at 1°C (33.8°F) to 10°C (50°F) for up to 14 days."
- For long-term storage, "skin should be maintained in a cryoprotectant under controlled cooling and freezing conditions. Freeze by cooling skin to at least –70°C (–94°F) at a rate of decline between 1°C (1.8°F) to 5°C (9°F) per minute. The skin can then be stored in a liquid nitrogen freezer."

Labeling the Tissue Specimen for Storage (AORN, 1992, *III*:21–1—21–2)

- Donor's name
- Donor's identification number
- Donor's pertinent medical information
- Donor's history
- Pathology report
- Culture and serologic testing reports
- Type and anatomic site of tissue
- Date and time of collection
- Method of collection
- Preservation solution and composition
- Recipient of the graft
- Recipient's identification number
- Date and time of transplantation
- Anatomic site of transplantation
- Informed consents from donor or donor's responsible party

Directing the Transfer of Cultures and Specimens to the Laboratory

- Ensure that the transporter understands where and to whom the culture or specimen is to be delivered.
- Ensure that assistive personnel responsible for transportation duties receive specific training on handling cultures and specimens during transportation.
- Training should focus on completion of the logbook, precautions to take if the specimen container is contaminated, and recognition and identification of laboratory slips.

Communicating Intraoperative Laboratory or Pathology Reports to the Surgeon

- The circulating nurse facilitates the communication of intraoperative laboratory or pathology reports between the surgeon and the laboratory or the pathology department.
- Direct communication between the surgeon and the laboratory technician or the pathologist is preferred.
- The technician or pathologist should be notified if the patient is awake for the procedure. If this is not possible, however, a written report should be presented to the surgeon.
- If the circulating nurse must serve as a conduit of oral communication, write the information, verify it for accuracy with the pathologist or the laboratory technician, and then give it to the surgeon.
- Attach written reports to the patient's record.

CRITICAL COMPETENCIES FOR THE REGISTERED NURSE FIRST ASSISTANT

This section provides a step-by-step discussion of how to
- Handle tissue with instruments
- Provide hemostasis
- Facilitate postoperative care

The content in this section is also intended for perioperative nurses who have limited their practice to the scrub and circulating nurse roles. Surgeon practice patterns are evolving, and more perioperative nurses will be called on to provide registered nurse first assistant (RNFA) services in the future. This section will provide the knowledge necessary for acquiring the skills and abilities to function as a first assistant.

HANDLING TISSUES WITH INSTRUMENTS

The RNFA demonstrates competency to handle tissues with instruments by
- Providing exposure during surgery
- Clamping tissue
- Grasping tissue
- Suturing
- Cutting tissue

Principles of Surgical Technique (Table 1)
Instrument Terminology
Categories of Surgical Instruments (Table 2)

TABLE 1
Principles of Surgical Technique

Plan the incision.

Make the skin incision with one stroke of evenly applied pressure on the scalpel.

Handle tissue carefully and as little as possible.

Provide hemostasis.

Preserve blood supply.
Débride necrotic and devitalized tissue.

Keep tissues moist.

Carefully and accurately approximate tissues.

Immobilize the wound.

Adapted from *Ethicon wound closure manual* (1988). (p. 5). Somerville, NJ: Ethicon, Inc.

Planning and designing the location, length, and depth of the incision achieves optimal exposure. Making the incision just long enough affords sufficient operating space while reducing the amount of tissue trauma. The direction of the incision may be a factor in wound healing. Wounds heal side to side, not end to end.

Making the skin incision with one stroke of evenly applied pressure on the scalpel aids in tissue approximation during wound closure. Sharp dissection cuts through other tissues. While cutting, watch for underlying nreves, blood vessels, and muscles in order to preserve as many as possible.

Carefully placed and handled retractors prevent undue pressure on tissues. Excessive pressure and tension on tissues impairs circulation of blood, slows lymph flow, alters the local physiologic state of the wound, and predisposes to microbial colonization. Reducing tissue trauma to a minimum aids the healing mechanisms of the body.

Hemostasis not only prevents loss of the patient's blood but also provides a field as bloodless as possible for accurate dissection. Bleeding may occur from transected or penetrated vessels, or there may be a diffuse oozing from large denuded surfaces. Mass ligation fo large areas of tissue may produce necrosis and prolong healing time. Complete hemostasis before closing the wound reduces the chance of hematoma formation. A hematoma or seroma in the incision prevents the direct apposition essential to the union of wound surfaces. These can act as a culture medium for microbial growth, leading to wound infection.

Preservation of the blood supply to the wound promotes optimal healing.

Adequate débridement of all necrotic and devitalized tissue and removal of inflicted foreign bodies promote healing, especially of traumatic wounds. Foreign bodies, such as dirt, metal, and glass, increase the probability of wound infection.

Periodic irrigation of the wound with warm normal saline solution or covering exposed surfaces with saline-moistened sponges or laparotomy tapes prevents drying of tissues during long procedures.

Approximation of tissues as nontraumatically as possible and with precision eliminates dead space and minimizes the potential for wound disruption. Evaluation of each patient and selection of the proper wound-closure materials for the particular surgical circumstance provides maximal opportunity for healing. Accurate approximation of tissue without tension or strangulation promotes healing.

Adequate immobilization of the approximated wound, but not necessarily the entire anatomic part, promotes efficient healing and minimal scar formation.

TABLE 2
Categories of Surgical Instruments

Category	Examples	Uses
Sharps	Scalpels Scissors Bone cutters Rongeurs Chisels Osteotomes Saws Curets Dermatomes	Designed to incise and dissect tissue and bone
Clamps	Hemostats (artery forceps) Vascular clamps Intestinal clamps	Designed to control bleeding and maintain hemostasis; may be used to grasp or retract tissue
Graspers	Tissue forceps Tenacula Rib approximators Sponge forceps Towel clips Needle holders	Used to grasp and hold tissue or bone for dissection or retraction or to assist in suturing
Retractors	Self-retaining Hand-held	Designed to provide the best exposure with minimal trauma to surrounding tissue
Other	Suction tubes Dilators	Designed to clear the operative field of fluids and to open or clear anatomic passages

Adapted from Groah, L. K. (1983). *Operating room nursing: The perioperative role* (pp. 283–287). Reston, Va: Reston Publishing.

Providing Exposure

Overly aggressive traction, although achieving good exposure, may cause injury to the patient. Thus the RNFA should approach the task of providing exposure from a nursing perspective.

- Assess the patient preoperatively and develop a plan of care that provides balanced traction to meet the exposure needs of the surgeon and protect the patient from injury.
- During the assessment focus on patient variables that affect the ability to provide exposure: age, height, weight, body build, and physical deformities or limitations.
- Review the planned surgical procedure to determine the stages of the procedure that require exposure, the type of tissue and the location of vascular or nerve structures, the presence of organs, and the types of instrument available for exposure.

- Intraoperatively, implement the plan and continually assess the operative site to determine the effectiveness of providing exposure.
- If variables change during the procedure, modify the plan.
- After surgery, assess the patient to determine the presence of injury related to the provision of exposure.

Stabilizing Anatomic Structures

Sponges

- Use laparotomy and 4 × 4 or 4 × 8 inch radiopaque sponges to stabilize and hold anatomic structures.
- Use wet or dry sponges to hold back tissue or push it out of the way, thus providing better exposure for the surgeon.
- Use radiopaque sponges, 4 × 4 or 4 × 8 inches, to grasp and hold tissue such as muscle, fascia, subcutaneous tissue, and skin.
- Use laparotomy sponges for grasping and holding internal organs such as the large and small intestines.
- When using sponges to move or hold anatomic structures, handle the tissue gently but with a firm touch.
- Use laparotomy sponges to pack the bowel. Before packing, moisten the sponges in warm normal saline. Keep track of the number of sponges used and thoroughly examine the cavity for retained sponges before closure.

Intestinal Bag

- Use an intestinal bag to keep the bowel moist, retain body heat, and protect the bowel from inadvertent abrasion during an extended procedure.
- Monitor the moisture content of the intestinal bag and the tissue integrity of the bowel. Maintain moisture content with a wet towel or a large laparotomy sponge.
- Prevent inadvertent strangulation of the bowel by supporting the bag. A stack of towels placed between the assistant and the patient aids in this process.

Impervious Stockinet

- Use an impervious stockinet to isolate an extremity.
- Use the stockinet to hold, reposition, or provide traction on the extremity during the procedure.

Tapes and Other Devices

- Use tapes, such as cotton cord ties, vessel loops, and Penrose drains to move or hold anatomic structures during surgery and permit a better view of the operative field.

- After the surgeon exposes the tissue and passes the tape around the tissue, the anatomic structure can be gently moved from the operative field.
- Exercise care when moving or holding a structure with a tape. Too much traction may tear the tissue. Apply the correct amount of traction in varying situations.

Suture Stitch

- Use a suture stitch to roll or hold tissue out of the way.
- After the stitch is in place, use it to apply the necessary traction.
- The stitch may also be attached to an instrument and the weight of the instrument used to apply the traction.
- The stitch can also be used to lift or hold tissue out of the operative field.

Using Retractors, Grasping Instruments, and Other Devices

- Hand-held or self-retaining retractors move and hold tissue and organs out of the operative field.
- Other instruments, such as clamps, stick sponges, and suction cannulas, push tissue and organs away from or pull them toward the surgeon, thus providing exposure of the operative field.
- Before using a retractor or any other device, assess the operative site. A misplaced retractor can compress, tear, or stretch blood vessels, nerves, and organs. The wrong type of grasping instrument can puncture delicate tissue, thus causing intraoperative and postoperative complications.
- Intraoperative assessment factors include the size and depth of the operative site, the physiologic status of the tissue, and the operative time.
- After placing retractors or using exposure devices, evaluate the tissue. If signs such as tissue blanching, cessation of pulse, or leaking of fluid appear, consider using other exposure methods.
- After surgery, if the patient complains of excessive musculoskeletal pain or neuromuscular impairment or has an unexplained fever, determine whether exposure techniques were too aggressive or whether an organ was inadvertently punctured.

Self-retaining Retractors

- Use self-retaining retractors to isolate and hold all types of tissue, from the most superficial to the deepest.
- To prevent tearing, use smooth self-retaining retractor blades on muscle.
- Use blades with sharp or dull teeth to hold fascia, subcutaneous tissue, and skin.

Hand-held Retractors

- Use hand-held retractors, such as Lahey goiter, Green goiter, Senn, U.S. Army, Mayo-Davis, and Volkmann retractors, to fine tune exposure.

Stick and Peanut Sponges

- Push tissue aside with stick sponges and peanut sponges (Kittner dissector sponges).
- Place stick sponges on straight or curved Foerster sponge forceps.
- Place peanut sponges on a Rochester-Péan clamp.
- The peanut sponge can be used as a tissue dissector.

Suction Devices

- Suction cannulas such as the Poole abdominal and Yankauer tonsil suction tubes may be used as exposure devices, especially if fluids need to be cleared.

Hand

- Use the hands for gently cupping, compressing, and pulling tissue and organs out of the way or into the line of sight.
- The hands allow controlled application of pressure and thus reduce the risk of tearing or puncturing the tissue or organ.

Countertraction Techniques

- Countertraction creates a plane of dissection that opens the connective tissue and provides exposure that gives the surgeon the necessary resistance during dissection of the organ or structure.

Clamping Tissue

- Use clamps to hold tissue in place.
- The hemostat is commonly used to grasp superficial vessels. When using a hemostat, place the thumb and middle finger (second long finger) inside the rings and hold the index finger against the hand for stabilization.
- Apply the hemostat so that the tip is as close as possible to the divided end of the vessel.
- After applying, remove the fingers from inside the rings and grasp the closed ring with the thumb and middle finger. When this position is obtained, gently and slightly lift and tilt the tip toward the surgeon.
- The index finger is then free to open the ratchet by applying pressure against the ring just as the surgeon increases the tension on the first knot.
- Next, the hemostat is carefully released and fully opened with a gradual, smooth motion.

Vascular Clamps

- After placing the clamp, hold it gently by the shank to avoid twisting or pulling.
- As with any hemostat, open the clamp widely before removing it to prevent drag on or accidental tears of the vessel.

Noncrushing Clamps

- During transection of the small bowel, place shodded intestinal clamps on a segment of the bowel to prevent spillage of enteric contents during the procedure.

Grasping Tissue

- When possible, lift tissue the fingers.
- Use forceps as an extension of the fingers.
- Grasp the forceps like a pencil and squeezed together by applying pressure with the thumb and index finger.
- Check forceps before surgery to see that they close precisely.
- Use smooth-jawed forceps on tissue that would likely bleed or easily perforate, such as bowel and liver.
- Use toothed forceps on skin, dense tissue, or scar tissue.
- During the surgery, use forceps to lift tissue and provide countertraction and stabilization.
- When selecting forceps, consider tissue sensitivity and its susceptibility to crushing.

Suturing

Principles of Suture Selection (Table 3)
Suture Materials (Table 4)

Needles

Needle Body Shapes and Typical Applications in Anatomic Sites and Tissues (Table 5)
Needle Points and Body Shapes With Typical Applications (Table 6)

Closure Methods

Primary Closure

- When doing a primary closure, bring each layer of tissue into correct approximation. This means that like tissues are brought together: fascia to fascia, muscle to muscle, subcutaneous tissue to subcutaneous tissue, and skin edges to skin edges.
- Approximation of like tissues and elimination of all dead space allow each layer to heal properly.
- Pulling the tissues together with the correct amount of tension is crucial for a successful closure. If sutures are too tight, the tissue

TABLE 3
Principles of Suture Selection

Principle	Rationale
When a wound has reached maximal strength, sutures are no longer needed.	Tissues that ordinarily heal slowly, such as skin, fascia, and tendons, should usually be closed with nonabsorbable sutures.
	Tissues that heal rapidly, such as stomach, colon, and bladder, may be closed with absorbable sutures.
Foreign bodies in potentially contaminated tissues may convert contamination to infection.	Avoid multifilament sutures, which may convert a contaminated wound into an infected one.
	Use monofilament or absorbable sutures in potentially contaminated tissues.
Where cosmetic results are important, close and prolonged apposition of wounds and avoidance of irritants will produce the best result.	Use the smallest inert monofilament suture materials, such as nylon or polypropylene.
	Avoid skin sutures and close subcuticularly whenever possible.
	Under certain circumstances, to secure close apposition of skin edges, skin-closure tape may be used.
Foreign bodies in the presence of fluids containing high concentrations of crystalloids may act as a nidus for precipitation and stone formation.	In the urinary and biliary tract, use rapidly absorbed sutures.
Selecting suture size.	Use the finest size, commensurate with the natural strength of the tissue.
	If the postoperative course of the patient may produce sudden strains on the suture line, reinforce it with retention sutures. Remove them as soon as the patient's condition is stabilized.

From *Ethicon wound closure manual* (1988). (p. 37–38). Somerville, NJ: Ethicon, Inc.

blanches and then strangulates, causing it to die for lack of an adequate blood supply.

- If sutures slip or become loose, dead space may form and fluid may seep into the wound, thus causing poor wound healing.

COMMON TECHNIQUES

- Use a continuous suture, also called a running stitch, to close a tissue layer by passing one strand of suture back and forth between the two edges of the wound (Table 7).
- An interrupted suture line is a series of singly placed stitches. As each suture is placed, it is tied and cut. The technique is used

TABLE 4
Suture Materials

Suture	Filament
Catgut	
Plain	
Chromic	
Polyglactin 910 (Vicryl)	Braided
Polydioxanone	Monofilament
Silk	Braided
Cotton	Twisted
Wire	Monofilament
Nylon	Monofilament
Polypropylene (Prolene)	Monofilament
Polyester fiber	
Mersilene	Braided
Ethibond	Braided

From Nora, P. F. (1991). *Operative surgery: Principles and techniques* (3rd ed). (p. 11). Philadelphia: W. B. Saunders.

Absorption	Uses
5–70 d	Ligature 3–0
	Ophthalmology
20–90 d	Gastrointestinal anastomoses 3–0, 4–0
	Fascia 0
	Skin, oral mucosa, genitourinary tract
	Ophthalmology
40–90 d	Ligature 3–0
	Fascia 0
	Subcutaneous tissue 3–0
	Peritoneum 2–0
	Urinary tract
	Microsurgery 8–0, 11–0
	Ophthalmology
90–200 d	Abdominal and thoracic closure
	Subcuticular
	Colorectal
	Orthopedic
Nonabsorbable	Ligature 3–0
	Gastrointestinal anastomoses 3–0
	Skin 4–0
	Blood vessel 5–0
Nonabsorbable	Fascia No. 30
	Subcutaneous tissue No. 50
	Skin No. 80
Nonabsorbable	Skin Nos. 34, 36
	Fascia Nos. 30, 32
	Retention No. 28
	Tendons
	Neurosurgery
	Orthopedic
Nonabsorbable	Skin 6–0, 5–0, 4–0
	Fascia 0
	Retention 0
	Microsurgery 8–0, 11–0
	Vascular
Nonabsorbable	Skin 6–0, 5–0, 4–0
	Fascia 0
	Retention 0
	Microsurgery 8–0, 11–0
	Vascular 6–0
	Tendons
	Ophthalmology
Nonabsorbable	Same as silk
Nonabsorbable	Same as silk

TABLE 5

Needle Body Shapes and Typical Applications in Anatomic Sites and Tissues

Shape	Typical Applications	
Straight	Gastrointestinal tract Nasal cavity Nerve Oral cavity	Pharynx Skin Tendon Vessels
Half-curved	Skin, rarely used	
1/4 circle	Eye, primary application Microsurgical procedures	
3/8 circle	Aponeurosis Biliary tract Dura Eye Fascia Gastrointestinal tract Muscle Myocardium	Nerve Perichondrium Periosteum Peritoneum Pleura Tendon Urogenital tract Vessels
1/2 circle	Biliary tract Eye Gastrointestinal tract Muscle Nasal cavity Oral cavity Pelvis	Peritoneum Pharynx Pleura Respiratory tract Skin Subcutaneous fat Urogenital tract
5/8 circle	Cardiovascular system Nasal cavity Oral cavity Pelvis Urogenital tract, primary application	
Compound Curved	Eye, anterior segment	

From *Ethicon wound closure manual* (1988). (p. 42). Somerville, NJ: Ethicon, Inc.

more often, even though it takes more time, because the integrity of the suture line remains intact if a suture breaks. In addition, if infection is present, microorganisms are less likely to travel along the primary suture line of interrupted stitches (Ethicon, 1988, p. 11).

Secondary Closure

- In the presence of an infection or gross contamination, use secondary closure. This allows access to the contaminated tissue for cleaning and enables the tissue to recover from the infection before final closure.
- During the first stage of a secondary closure, close the deep tissue, such as the peritoneum and fascia, with a monofilament suture material. Leave the next tissue layers open to permit irrigation of the wound and instillation of antibiotics during dressing changes.
- Some surgeons insert skin sutures during a secondary closure. This technique allows the incision edges to pull together, thus reducing the amount of tension placed on the incision. The amount of scar tissue that forms from this type of closure is also decreased. One should place the skin sutures far apart to allow the proper healing process.

Retention Sutures

- In the presence of gross contamination, obesity, tissue loss, or excessive tissue damage such as the type seen with massive trauma, the surgeon may use retention sutures. Approximating the incision or damaged tissue with a large through-and-through nonabsorbable suture material reduces tension and holds incision edges together until healing is complete.
- Place retention sutures about 2 inches away from each edge of the wound. When placing the retention sutures, select one of the following closure techniques: through-and-through retention sutures or buried coaptation-retention sutures (Ethicon, 1988, p. 12).

THROUGH-AND-THROUGH RETENTION SUTURES
- Insert through-and-through retention sutures before the peritoneum is closed.
- Place through-and-through sutures from inside the peritoneal cavity by inserting the suture through the peritoneum, all abdominal layers, and the skin with a simple interrupted or figure-of-eight stitch.
- Next, close the wound in layers for a distance of about three-fourths the length of the wound.
- Draw the retention sutures together and tie them. While tying, place a finger in the abdominal cavity to prevent strangulation of

TABLE **6**

Needle Points and Body Shapes With Typical Applications in Anatomic Sites and Tissues

Shape	Typical Applications
Conventional Cutting	Ligament Nasal cavity Oral cavity Pharynx Skin Tendon
Reverse Cutting	Fascia Ligament Nasal cavity Oral mucosa Skin Tendon sheath
MICRO-POINT. Reverse Cutting Needle	Eye
Precision Point Cutting	Plastic or cosmetic procedures Skin
Side-cutting Spatulated	Eye, primary application Microsurgical procedures Reconstructive ophthalmic procedures

From *Ethicon wound closure manual* (1988). (p. 73). Somerville, NJ: Ethicon, Inc.

Shape	Typical Applications
POINT TAPERCUT. Surgical Needle BODY	Bronchus Calcified tissue Fascia Ligament Nasal cavity Oral cavity Ovary Perichondrium Periosteum Pharynx Tendon Trachea Uterus Vessels, sclerotic
POINT Taper BODY	Aponeurosis Biliary tract Dura Fascia Gastrointestinal tract Muscle Myocardium Nerve Peritoneum Pleura Subcutaneous fat Urogenital tract Vessels
POINT Blunt BODY	Blunt dissection through friable tissue Kidney Liver Spleen Uterine cervix for ligating incompetent cervix

TABLE 7
Commonly Used Stitches

Continuous Suture	Interrupted Sutures
To Appose Skin and Other Tissue	
Over-and-over	Over-and-over
Vertical mattress	Vertical mattress
Horizontal mattress	Horizontal mattress
Subcuticular	
To Invert Tissue	
Lembert	Lembert
Cushing	Halsted
Connell	Pursestring
To Evert Tissue	
Horizontal mattress	Horizontal mattress

From *Ethicon wound closure manual* (1988). (p. 13). Somerville, NJ: Ethicon, Inc.

the viscera during closure. Closure of the remainder of the wound continues in a similar manner (Ethicon, 1988, p. 12).

BURIED COAPTATION-RETENTION SUTURES

- Insert buried coaptation-retention sutures after the peritoneum is closed.
- Place the suture through the fascia and then the skin.
- These retention sutures are placed "approximately two centimeters apart in the posterior rectus sheath and peritoneum in the so-called 'far-and-near' or 'far-near-near-far' fashion."
- After inserting the retention sutures, close the wound in layers and then tie the retention sutures (Ethicon, 1988, p. 12).

Use of the Needle Holder

- When passing a needle holder, the scrub nurse should place it firmly and with feeling in the palm of the assistant's hand.
- To prevent dragging of the suture across the sterile field, the scrub nurse holds the suture (Ethicon, 1988, p. 51).
- After receiving the needle holder from the scrub nurse, grasp it firmly and insert the thumb and fourth finger (ring finger) through the rings of the instrument. This technique enables the RNFA to use the index and middle fingers to control and push the needle through the tissue.
- When inserting the needle, rotate the wrist, thus pushing the needle through the tissue with one smooth easy motion.
- Palming is another way to handle a needle holder. With this technique, the RNFA places only the fourth finger through the

ring of the instrument, which permits opening and closing of the needle holder without having to place the thumb into the ring. Many prefer this technique because it allows the assistant to handle the needle holder more quickly.

LOADING OF THE NEEDLE HOLDER

- Correct placement of the needle in the needle holder prevents it from turning when it enters the tissue during suturing.
- Place the needle in the jaws just below the point where it flattens out.

Placement of Sutures

- When inserting the needle, place the point at a right angle to the tissue. This technique allows the needle a clean and smooth entry through the tissue.
- After inserting the needle, release it, grasp down from the point, and pull it through.
- Unless there is no other way to pull the needle through the tissue, avoid grasping the point.
- Getting the needle and suture through both sides of the incision usually requires two motions. Therefore, after pulling the needle through one side, reposition it in the needle holder and place the point in the tissue so that it exits the tissue at a right angle.
- To bring the incision edges properly together, keep the suture at the same level in the tissue.
- Next, advance the suture through the tissue by using a smooth, uninterrupted, and gentle pulling motion.
- When suturing, bring like tissues together: peritoneum to peritoneum, muscle to muscle, fascia to fascia, subcutaneous tissue to subcutaneous tissue, and skin to skin. Many surgeons use the Smead-Jones stitch when closing the abdomen.
- When suturing, the free end of the suture is easily contaminated if not controlled. Control the free end by placing the suture to the right of the needle holder when using the right hand and to the left when using the left hand.
- When using a straight needle for closure, grasp the skin edges gently but firmly with a tissue forceps. Lifting the edge of the incision aids in placing the needle point in the tissue.
- After the needle is through one side, repeat the procedure with the opposite incision edge.
- Place the suture at an equal depth and distance from the skin edges.
- If not actually performing the closure, handle the ends of the suture during closure. Prevent knots and redundant suture from getting in the way of the surgeon by keeping the suture taut and straight.

- Help control the tissue by placing tension on the suture. This maneuver not only makes placement of the next suture easier but also provides the necessary exposure for the surgery to proceed smoothly.

Staples

BASIC REQUIREMENT FOR APPOSING SKIN WITH STAPLES
- The edges of the cuticular and subcuticular layers are everted, that is, aligned with the edges slightly raised in an outward direction. As it heals, the tissue will tend to flatten out and form an even surface.
- The skin edges must be aligned as close to their original configuration on the horizontal plane as possible. If one edge is allowed to slide or to be placed in a location other than its original one, the best cosmetic results will not be obtained and unnecessary scars can form (Ethicon, 1988, p. 57).

PLACING STAPLES
- Before placing the skin staples, force the skin edges together with one tissue forceps until the edges evert or pick up each wound edge individually with two tissue forceps and approximate the edges.
- Next, tension is applied to either end of the incision until the tissue edges begin to approximate each other (Ethicon, 1988, p. 57).

Surgical Knots

- When suturing, use the simple or overhand knot, square knot, granny knot, and surgeons' knot.
- The simple knot is the first step of basic knot tying, whereas the square knot is a complete and true knot.
- Unless requested by the surgeon, avoid the granny knot. This slip knot does not provide the security necessary to ensure that tissue holds together and vessels remain closed.
- Maintain tension or traction on the tissue with the surgeons' knot. This knot does not slip after the first throw is in place.
- Use the square knot because it provides a secure and competent knot in or around the tissue.
- An area that requires a deep tie may also need a suture ligature.
- After the surgeon places a suture ligature, the knot is tied by the same process as described above.
- After insertion of the suture ligature, the suture is brought back to the opposite side of the hemostat and the knot is completed.
- When making a deep tie, use a needle holder to complete the tie.
- Loop the suture around the end of the holder, grasp the other end of the suture, and pull it through the loop; this starts the

knot. To complete the knot, wrap in the opposite direction to form a square knot.

Applying Knot Tension

- Securing the knot prevents it from falling out of the tissue. Use of the correct amount of tension when tying the knot prevents slipping when the final knot is in place.
- The knot tension holds the tissue together and keeps the vessel closed. This tension should approximate, not strangulate or tear, the tissue.
- Maintain firm and steady tension during knot tying by holding one end of the suture still while tying the knot. Steady tension prevents the suture material from breaking during the tie. Jerking, sawing, or snapping the suture may cause it to break during the procedure.
- Because tissues swell when knots are placed, use only the necessary number of throws to complete the knot. This reduces the bulk of the suture left in the patient. When tying deep knots, to ensure proper placement of the tie on the tissue, always carry the suture down to the tissue with the tip of the finger.
- Keeping the vessel closed or the tissue in place necessitates properly placed, firmly set, and squared knots. Different types of tissue require different amounts of tension to provide the correct closure. If the tension is too loose, the incision gaps. If the tension is too tight, the tissue strangulates, thus creating the potential for necrosis.

Cutting of Sutures

- When cutting sutures, run the tip of the scissors down the length of the suture strand to the knot. If surgical gut has been used, cut the strand 6 mm from the knot.
- Cut synthetic sutures 3 mm from the knot to minimize the amount of foreign material left in the wound.
- Before cutting the suture, ensure that the tips of the scissors are in sight to avoid cutting tissue.
- As sutures are cut, remove the ends from the operative site (Ethicon, 1988, p. 14).

Cutting Tissue

Scalpels

- Change the blade as soon as it becomes dull, because the edge must be sharp and smooth.
- The type of operation and the patient's size determine not only the size and location of the initial incision but the type of blade as well.

- For large incisions, the scalpel handle is held against the palm with the thumb and fingers gripping it from above. This is known as the power grip.
- Hold the blade vertical to the skin to prevent beveling and cut the dermis and epidermis quickly with a single stroke, applying even pressure. This technique promotes precision approximation of skin, which promotes wound healing.
- Control the depth of the incision by downward pressure of the index finger. A wide blade such as the No. 10 or 20 is commonly used.
- Use the No. 15 blade for small incisions and for dissecting fine tissue. This blade can also be used with a pencil-like grip.
- Use the No. 11 blade to make a small skin incision. This blade is often used to puncture an abscess, cut a vessel wall, or make a sharp cut in a small structure such as the fallopian tube.
- Use the crescent-shaped No. 12 blade in a hole when the surgeon may impale tissue with the tip as she or he cuts it.

Scissors

- Use scissors for dissecting tissue, severing clamped blood vessels, and cutting suture.
- When using scissors, maintain control by inserting the thumb and fourth (ring) finger through the handle rings. The index and middle fingers are then used to stabilize the scissors as it cuts.

PROVIDING HEMOSTASIS

The RNFA demonstrates competency to provide hemostasis by

- Recognizing alterations in clotting mechanisms that put the patient at risk for experiencing intraoperative and postoperative bleeding
- Recognizing hypovolemic shock
- Applying mechanical methods to control bleeding
- Applying thermal methods to control bleeding
- Applying chemical methods to control bleeding

Recognizing Hypovolemic Shock
Stages of Hypovolemic Shock (Table 8)

MILD SHOCK (loss of 20% or less of blood volume)

- Determine whether the patient has poor skin perfusion, especially on the feet, which may be pale, cool, and clammy. The subcutaneous veins on the foot collapse. (Skin pallor due to vasoconstriction is the first sign of hypovolemia. However, although skin pallor is a sensitive physical sign, it is nonspecific. Fear, hypothermia, and hypoglycemia also produce poor skin perfusion.)

TABLE **8**
Stages of Hypovolemic Shock

Peripheral venous constriction	Trunk cooling
Poor capillary filling	Agitation
Pallor	Decreased pain sensation
Peripheral cooling	Loss of deep tendon reflexes
Oliguria	Acidotic breathing
Increased pulse rate	Deep pallor
Thirst	Loss of consciousness
Increased respiratory rate	Death
Hypotension	

From Polk, H. S., Stone, H. H., Gardener, B. (eds) (1987). *Basic surgery* (3rd ed).
(p. 56). East Norwalk, Conn: Appleton-Century-Crofts.

- Check the patient's blood pressure. If the patient is in a supine position, the blood pressure and pulse remain normal. When the patient sits or stands rapidly, however, the blood pressure falls and the pulse rate rises.
- Check the patient's urine output. In mild shock, output is normal.
- The patient may complain of being cold or thirsty.
MODERATE SHOCK (loss of 20% to 40% of circulating volume)
- Look for pale skin and a low urine output.
- Check the patient's blood pressure. Many patients maintain a normal blood pressure and pulse in a supine position. A few, however, have a drop in pressure and a rise in pulse rate.
SEVERE SHOCK (loss of 40% or more of the circulating volume)
- Look for hypotension, oliguria, and tachycardia. These are indicators of severe shock.
- Check the patient's skin perfusion. It will be poor, and as the hypovolemia worsens or persists, the patient will show changes in the electrocardiogram (an indication of myocardial ischemia).
- Observe the patient's mental status. As circulation decreases to the brain, the patient may become agitated, restless, or obtunded.

Assessing the Patient's Clotting Mechanisms

- Before surgery, assess the patient's clotting mechanisms.
- When a patient's history or physical examination suggests bleeding or clotting difficulties, the physician orders platelet and coagulation studies.
- If no studies have been obtained on these patients, recommend appropriate tests: platelet count, prothrombin time (PT), partial thromboplastin time (PTT), thrombin time, quantitative platelet counts, and bleeding time.

- Compare coagulation study results to the control study results. (Quantitative platelet counts less than 60,000/mm^3 indicate that the patient may have an occult thrombocytopenia, either acquired or congenital. A lack of platelets prolongs bleeding time [Polk et al., 1987].)
- Suspect qualitative platelet defects if the patient takes antiplatelet drugs. For example, aspirin prolongs bleeding time, an effect that can last up to 3 to 5 days.
- Determine whether the patient takes other drugs, besides aspirin, that have antiplatelet action such as dipyridamole (Persantine), sulfinpyrazone (Anturane), nonsteroidal anti-inflammatory drugs (sulindac [Clinoril], ibuprofen [Motrin], piroxicam [Feldene]), and antihistamines, which also have antiplatelet action.
- Since high doses of dextran also cause qualitative platelet abnormalities, determine whether the patient has received dextran.
- Assess the patient's renal function. Patients with renal failure are at risk because qualitative platelet abnormalities increase proportionately with the degree of uremia.
- Look for other conditions, such as myeloproliferative diseases, and check for incidents of bone marrow replacement. These patients may experience qualitative platelet abnormalities (Polk et al., 1987).
- Check for acquired bleeding disorders such as cirrhosis and hepatitis. These disorders impair clotting factors, especially vitamin K–dependent factors.
- Look for conditions that may result in vitamin K depletion such as malnutrition, obstructive jaundice, antibiotic sterilization of the gastrointestinal tract, or malabsorption such as ulcerative colitis or Crohn's disease. In such cases, the patient has a prolonged PT and PTT.
- In the event of a vitamin K deficiency, alert the surgeon. Parenteral administration of vitamin K can improve clotting times in 8 to 12 hours. (In the presence of liver disease the degree to which vitamin K the patient should take depends on the extent of parenchymal cell damage [Guyton, 1991].)
- During the preoperative assessment, note whether the patient takes anticoagulant drugs such as coumarin compounds (sodium warfarin [Coumadin]). These drugs, although they have no anticoagulating effect in vitro, work by inhibiting the synthesis of vitamin K–dependent factors and prothrombin (Polk et al., 1987).
- During the preoperative assessment, identify patients at risk for disseminated intravascular coagulation. (Risk factors for disseminated intravascular coagulation include widespread metastatic

disease, massive trauma or burns, gram-negative or gram-positive sepsis, some viral and malarial infections, exposure to incompatible blood products, retroplacental hemorrhage, and snake bites [Polk et al., 1987].)

Controlling Bleeding by Mechanical Methods
Pressure
PRESSURE TECHNIQUES
- Apply direct pressure with one or more fingers to the site of bleeding.
- When applying indirect pressure, use the fingers or the palm of the hand to compress the area adjacent to the site of active bleeding.
- Use laparotomy sponges or other materials, such as a pack, to apply pressure.

SUPPLIES
- Dry laparotomy sponges or other suitable packing materials

INTERVENTIONS
- Before using pressure, assess the need for hemostasis and determine the appropriateness of using pressure on the anatomic structure requiring hemostasis.
- After the skin is incised, apply moderate pressure all along the incised surface.
- Control subcutaneous bleeding with a dry laparotomy sponge. Place the sponge on the bleeding surface and press with the fingertips; this provides hemostasis and countertraction. The surgeon often does the same on the opposite surface.
- If necessary, use two dry laparotomy sponges, one for each side of the wound, and pull on both sides of the incised surface in opposite directions.
- Use a dry laparotomy sponge to apply direct digital pressure to the area of active bleeding.
- If the site of bleeding is hidden from view or if direct pressure is unsuccessful or is impractical, apply indirect pressure or pressure to adjacent structures.
- For sudden and profuse bleeding, apply direct digital pressure. Exert only enough pressure to stop or slow the blood flow. Use pressure as a temporary measure until bleeding is controlled by other means, such as ligatures and clips.
- Inform the scrub nurse and the circulating nurse of the location and number of laparotomy sponges used as packs. Report when the sponges are removed. Use only radiopaque packing materials.
- Before closing the wound, recheck areas that were packed for hemostasis.

Hemostatic Clips

- Use hemostatic clips to ligate blood vessels.

SUPPLIES AND EQUIPMENT

- Tissue forceps
- Clip appliers
- Clips

INTERVENTIONS

- Before using clips, assess the need for hemostasis and determine the appropriateness of using the clips on the anatomic structure requiring hemostasis.
- Check clip appliers to ensure proper functioning. Look for symmetrical jaws that securely hold the clip and close without overlapping.
- In the event of bleeding, isolate the severed vessel and apply direct digital pressure with a dry laparotomy sponge to control bleeding.
- Next, slowly roll the sponge off the incised vessel and grasp it with a nontraumatic tissue forceps.
- Apply the clip to a skeletonized vessel.
- Avoid clipping the tissue surrounding the vessel.
- After skeletonizing a vessel, apply two clips and then cut the vessel between the clips. Avoid clipping the tissue surrounding the vessel.

Controlling Bleeding by Thermal Methods

Electrocautery

- Follow institutional protocols regarding electrosurgical unit (ESU) safety and apply the AORN recommendations for electrocautery (AORN, 1992).
- After positioning the patient so that the skin has no contact with metal, apply the dispersive electrode to clean, dry skin over a large muscle mass.
- Place the electrode as close to the operative site as feasible.
- Avoid bony prominences, hairy surfaces, scarred areas, implanted metal devices, or prostheses.
- Ensure that the pad has even contact with the skin.
- Check all connections to ensure that they are intact.
- Repeat the inspection whenever the patient's position is changed.
- Set the ESU to the operator's specifications. Confirm settings verbally with the operator.
- Keep settings at the lowest levels possible.
- Use isolated electrocardiographic leads and do not place the leads between the operative site and the dispersive electrode.

- Before using the ESU, assess the need for hemostasis and determine the appropriateness of using the instrument on the anatomic structure requiring hemostasis by evaluating vessel size. If the vessel is large, use a ligature or clips to control the bleeding.
- Check the active electrode (pencil) before use. Look for frayed cords and ensure that the tip of the active electrode is securely seated.
- Activate the electrode by depressing and then releasing the appropriate switches. The unit should activate immediately when the switch is depressed and deactivate when the switch is released.
- Do not indiscriminately activate the electrode.
- Identify the cautery site and adjacent structures. Do not cauterize adjacent nerves or tissue unless their destruction is intended.
- In the event of bleeding, isolate the severed vessel and apply direct digital pressure with a dry laparotomy sponge to control bleeding. Next, slowly roll the sponge off the severed vessel and touch the vessel with the activated electrode for as long as it takes to blanch the tissue. Charring the tissue is usually not necessary.
- When using tissue forceps, grasp the end of the vessel with the forceps and touch the activated electrode to the tissue forceps for as long as it takes to blanch the tissue.
- Avoid grasping the surrounding tissue with the forceps.
- If the scrub nurse operates the active electrode, verbally indicate when to begin the electrical current.
- Stop the flow of current by releasing the tissue from the grasp of the forceps.

Laser (AORN, 1992, *III*:10–1—10–3)

- Cooperate with the circulator in applying the AORN recommendations for laser use in the operating room (AORN, 1992) when preparing the room, the surgical team, and the patient for laser surgery.
- Place warning signs at all entrances to the room.
- Wear eye protection appropriate to the laser being used.
- Place appropriate eyewear on closed eyelids of the anesthetized patient or provide eye protection if the patient is awake.
- Apply damp laparotomy sponges to the tissue surrounding the operative site.
- Use flame-resistant or moistened drapes.
- Use nonreflective instruments near the site of laser use.
- Use wet tongue blades or quartz or titanium rods as a backstop for the beam. This prevents the beam from inadvertently hitting underlying tissue.

- Inform the circulator when the laser is not in use so that she or he may set the laser on standby.
- Evacuate the noxious fumes and laser plume with appropriate scavenging devices.

Plasma Scalpel

- Before using the plasma scalpel, assess the need for hemostasis and determine the appropriateness of using the instrument on the anatomic structure requiring hemostasis.
- Request the appropriate temperature settings (110°C for skin incisions). For other tissues, the temperature setting is usually between 180°C and 240°C).
- Maintain a dry operative field by blotting blood and other body fluids with dry laparotomy sponges.
- When using the blade, make long slow strokes to prevent the onset of bleeding. Blood vessels 2 mm and smaller should seal as they are cut. For larger vessels, exert light pressure on the bleeder with the flat of the blade.
- During the procedure, occasionally clean the blade with a dry laparotomy sponge to prevent thermal isolation.
- Do not allow an activated electrocautery tip to come in contact with the blade.
- Do not use the heated blade to make skin incisions through plastic adhesive drapes.
- Do not rest the blade on the drapes or on the patient when activated.
- Do not immerse the handle in liquid.

Documentation and Communication Procedures

ELECTROCAUTERY
- Generator number
- Power settings
- Electrocardiographic electrode and dispersive plate placement
- Condition of the skin at the site of the dispersive plate and electrocardiographic electrodes before and after the procedure
- Note any postoperative skin lesions that were not apparent preoperatively.

LASER
- Unit number
- Power setting
- Safety precautions used
- Describe preoperative and postoperative condition of the skin surrounding the operative site.

PLASMA SCALPEL
- Number of the power unit
- Note the presence of thermal burns, if they occur

Controlling Bleeding by Chemical Methods
Supplies and Equipment
- Straight Mayo scissors
- Dry tissue forceps free from blood
- Dry laparotomy sponges
- Suction

Microfibrillar Collagen Hemostat
- Do not sterilize microfibrillar collagen hemostat. It is inactivated by autoclaving, and use of ethylene oxide is contraindicated.
- Ensure that surfaces are dry. Microfibrillar collagen hemostat adheres to wet gloves, instruments, and tissue surfaces.
- Do not moisten microfibrillar collagen hemostat with saline solution or thrombin. These agents impair its ability to act as a hemostatic agent.
- Do not use in the presence of systemic disorders. Microfibrillar collagen hemostat cannot control bleeding that is due to systemic disorders.
- Assess the need for the use of microfibrillar collagen hemostat to provide hemostasis
- Ascertain whether the patient has any known allergies to bovine derivatives.
- Determine the adequacy of primary efforts at hemostasis (clamping, electrocautery, tying, and suturing) before using microfibrillar collagen hemostat. Evaluate the rate of blood flow. Ascertain whether the bleeding site can be made visible and accessible.
- Determine the appropriateness of microfibrillar collagen hemostat to the anatomic structure on which it would be used.
- Keep microfibrillar collagen hemostat away from skin edges when closing the incision.
- Do not use microfibrillar collagen hemostat on bone surfaces to which prosthetic devices are to be attached with methyl methacrylate.
- Determine the appropriateness of microfibrillar collagen hemostat in light of the wound classification. Use of microfibrillar collagen hemostat in the presence of contaminated or infected wounds is ill advised.
- When applying or assisting in the application of microfibrillar collagen hemostat, suction or sponge the area dry. Provide additional exposure as needed.
- With clean, dry tissue forceps, such as Mayo forceps, apply microfibrillar collagen hemostat to the bleeding site.
- Using moderate pressure, hold a dry lap sponge on the bleeding site. Hemostasis usually occurs in about 1 minute. The time will vary, depending on the force and severity of the bleeding. Three

to 5 minutes may be required to stop brisk bleeding, such as that from splenic lacerations or arterial suture lines.

- Use additional microfibrillar collagen hemostat as needed.
- Apply the nonwoven web form of microfibrillar collagen hemostat in small squares to the bleeding site.
- Cover the site with a dry cottonoid for small areas or a lap sponge for larger areas.
- A suction tip may be used to hold pressure on the cottonoid. Pack microfibrillar collagen hemostat firmly into the spongy bone surface to control oozing from cancellous bone.
- Avoid spilling microfibrillar collagen hemostat on nonbleeding surfaces, particularly in the abdominal or thoracic viscera.
- Remove excess microfibrillar collagen hemostat from all surfaces by gently teasing with blunt forceps and irrigation before closing the wound.
- Avoid the reintroduction of blood from operative sites treated with microfibrillar collagen hemostat. Notify the circulating nurse to discontinue the use of blood-scavenging equipment once microfibrillar collagen hemostat is used.
- Discard unused microfibrillar collagen hemostat.
- Do not resterilize microfibrillar collagen hemostat.

Absorbable Gelatin Sponge

- Heating gelatin sponge, however, affects absorption time (*Physician's Desk Reference,* 1992).
- Do not use on skin edges. Gelatin sponge interferes with the healing of the skin edges when used in the closure of incisions and has caused excessive fibrosis when used during tendon repairs.
- Do not use in the presence of inflammation. Adverse effects have occurred when gelatin sponge was used in areas of intense inflammation (*Physician's Desk Reference,* 1992).
- Determine the appropriateness of using gelatin sponge on the anatomic structure requiring hemostasis.
- Evaluate the appropriateness of the gelatin sponge on the basis of the wound classification.
- Gelatin sponge absorbs fluid, expands, and exerts pressure on adjacent structures. Therefore, do not use during neurosurgery, for tendon repairs, and in the presence of inflammation. Recommend the use of another agent.
- Before using gelatin sponge, evaluate the effectiveness of hemostasis by mechanical and thermal methods. Look at the rate of blood flow and, if possible, make the site accessible by clearing away blood with suction or a dry sponge.
- Provide additional exposure as needed.
- Cut pieces of gelatin sponges into the desired size.

- For dry application, compress each piece between the fingers and then use a clean tissue forceps to apply it to the bleeding site. Using moderate pressure, hold it with a dry laparotomy sponge on the bleeding site for 10 to 15 seconds.
- Apply a wet or damp piece. For wet application, the scrub nurse should have the sponges prepared for use by immersing the cut pieces in saline solution, squeezing out the air bubbles, and then placing the pieces back in the saline solution until used. For damp application, blot the piece of gelatin sponge on a dry laparotomy sponge. Using moderate pressure, hold the gelatin sponge in place with a dry laparotomy sponge for at least 10 to 15 seconds. Capillary action draws the blood into the gelatin. Wet the laparotomy sponge with saline solution to avoid pulling the gelatin off the site when removing the sponge.
- An alternative method of using wet or dry gelatin sponge is to apply suction to the laparotomy sponge while holding the gelatin in place. This technique draws blood into the gelatin and seems to hasten clotting.
- Pack gelatin loosely in closed spaces or cavities because it swells as it absorbs fluid. Apply light pressure in cavities or closed spaces.
- To prevent recurrent bleeding, leave the gelatin sponge in place. If desired, close the wound with the gelatin sponge left in place.
- Keep gelatin away from skin edges when closing the incision; gelatin interferes with wound healing.
- Discard unused gelatin sponges; do not resterilize.

Absorbable Collagen Sponge

- Before surgery, determine whether the patient has allergies to collagen sponges or bovine derivatives.
- Determine the appropriateness of using collagen sponge on the anatomic structure requiring hemostasis. In addition, evaluate the appropriateness of the collagen sponge on the basis of the wound classification. Avoid the use of collagen sponges in neurologic, urologic, and ophthalmologic procedures and in the presence of methyl methacrylate.
- Before using collagen sponge, evaluate the effectiveness of hemostasis by mechanical and thermal methods. Look at the rate of blood flow and, if possible, make the site accessible by clearing away blood with suction or a dry sponge.
- Provide additional exposure as needed.
- Pack collagen loosely in closed spaces or cavities because it swells as it absorbs fluid. Compression of adjacent structures can occur as the collagen swells. Do not use collagen sponges on bone surfaces to which prosthetic devices are to be attached with methyl methacrylate.

- Cut pieces of collagen sponges into the desired sizes. It is most effective when used dry. With clean tissue forceps, apply collagen sponge to the bleeding site. Hold it with a dry lap sponge on the bleeding site, using moderate pressure. Hemostasis usually occurs in 2 to 5 minutes. Remove excessive collagen before closing the wound.
- Keep collagen away from skin edges when closing the incision.
- Discard unused gelatin sponges and do not resterilize.

Oxidized Regenerated Cellulose

- Determine the appropriateness of using oxidized cellulose on the anatomic structure requiring hemostasis. In addition, evaluate the appropriateness of the oxidized cellulose on the basis of the wound classification.
- Before using oxidized cellulose, evaluate the effectiveness of hemostasis by mechanical and thermal methods. Look at the rate of blood flow and, if possible, make the site accessible by clearing away blood with suction or a dry sponge.
- Provide additional exposure as needed.
- Avoid use of oxidized cellulose in fractured bones, as it may interfere with callus formation.
- Avoid wrapping structures such as blood vessels and ureters.
- Cut pieces of oxidized cellulose into the desired size.
- Use only the amount necessary to achieve hemostasis.
- Apply oxidized cellulose dry, with clean tissue forceps, to the bleeding site. Hold it with a dry laparotomy sponge on the bleeding site, using moderate pressure until hemostasis is achieved.
- If possible, remove oxidized cellulose before closing the wound. It may, however, be left in place with no adverse effects if it is properly applied and is present in small amounts.
- Do not use oxidized cellulose as a packing material for bleeding wounds.
- Discard unused oxidized cellulose and do not resterilize.
- Evaluate the patient postoperatively for signs of stinging and burning, sneezing, or headaches when oxidized cellulose was used for epistaxis. Look for postoperative burning or stinging when oxidized cellulose was used after the removal of a nasal polyp or hemorrhoidectomy and applied to wound surfaces such as donor sites, venous stasis ulcerations, and dermabrasions. If it is causing the patient difficulty, recommend removal.

Documentation and Communication Procedures

- Document the use of microfibrillar collagen hemostat, gelatin sponge, collagen sponge, and oxidized cellulose in the intraoperative nurse's notes.

• Inform postoperative nurses if oxidized cellulose is used for packing or is applied to wound surfaces.

FACILITATING POSTOPERATIVE CARE

The RNFA demonstrates competency to facilitate postoperative care by
• Recognizing postoperative wound complications
• Recognizing fever, tachycardia, pulmonary complications, thrombophlebitis, urinary tract infections, and adynamic ileus
• Assessing postoperative comfort level
• Assessing nausea and vomiting
• Ensuring the proper functioning of devices employed to assist recovery

Considerations

• Critical variables that affect convalescence:
  1. Preoperative condition
  2. Operative time
  3. Amount of blood transfused
  4. Organ system involved in surgery
• Providing information to the PACU nurse:
  1. Facts about the patient's medical, social, and psychological history
  2. Type of surgery
  3. Pertinent intraoperative events
  4. Type of drugs administered during surgery
  5. The surgeon's postoperative orders (Table 9)

TABLE **9**
Routine Postoperative Orders

Activity—ambulation, bathroom privileges, and so on
Vital signs—if other than routine
Diet—nothing by mouth or specific diet
Intravenous fluids
Medications
   Pain
   Nausea
   Patient's regular medications
   Antibiotics
Drain or tube care
Input and output—provision for insertion of catheter if needed
Postoperative diagnostic studies—blood work, procedures, and so on

Adapted from Polk, H. S., Stone, H. H., Gardener, B. (eds) (1987). *Basic surgery* (3rd ed). (p. 7). East Norwalk, Conn: Appleton-Century-Crofts.

- Visiting the patient after surgery to
  1. Review vital signs and documentation of intake and output
  2. Check the functioning of devices used to help the patient's recovery
  3. Auscultate the heart, lungs, and abdomen
  4. Assess the legs for phlebitis
  5. Evaluate the progress of wound healing
  6. Record observations and refer for medical treatment as needed
- During daily visits look for signs of early postoperative complications and initiate treatment or referral before complications are exacerbated and critically affect the patient's postoperative course.

Wound Healing
Stages of Surgical Wound Healing (Table 10)
Risk Factors Affecting Wound Healing (Table 11)
Drugs That Delay Wound Healing (Table 12)
Typical Appearance Times of Complications After Major Abdominal Surgery (Table 13)

Recognizing Postoperative Wound Complications
Wound Infection (Table 14)
- Pain and tenderness due to irritation of local nerve endings
- Increased temperature of the area involved
- Redness in response to the vascularization process

TABLE **10**

Stages of Surgical Wound Healing

Stage	Time	Event	Cells
Inflammation (0–4 d)	0–2 h	Hemostasis	Platelets Erythrocytes Leukocytes
	0–4 d	Phagocytosis	Neutrophils Macrophages
Proliferation (2–22 d)	1–4 d	Epithelialization	Keratinocytes
	2–7 d	Neovascularization	Endothelial cells
	2–22 d	Collagen synthesis	Fibroblasts
	2–20 d	Contraction	Myofibroblasts
Maturation (21 d–2 y)		Collagen remodeling	Fibroblasts

Reprinted with permission from *AORN Journal*, Vol 49, p 506, February 1989. Copyright © AORN Inc, 10170 East Mississippi Avenue, Denver, CO, 80231.

- Swelling due to edema and inflammatory exudate
- Wound complications frequently have systemic manifestations, such as elevated temperature and tachycardia. A clue to the type of pathogen involved is the postoperative day on which the infection becomes apparent.

TABLE **11**
Risk Factors Affecting Wound Healing

Systemic	Trauma
Age	Underlying pathologic condition
Smoking	(diabetes, cancer)
Obesity	Prolonged surgery (>3 h)
Stress	Night or emergency surgery
Anemia	
Uremia	*Local*
Hypovolemia	Surgical technique
Hypoxia	Blood supply to wound
Malnutrition	Mechanical stress
Protein deficiency	Suture materials
Vitamin deficiency (vitamins C,	Suturing techniques
A, B, and K)	Radiation
Mineral deficiency (zinc, copper,	Infection
magnesium)	Oxygen tension
Drugs	Antiseptics
Corticosteroids	Presence of drain
Chemotherapeutic agents	Preparation of operative site
Length of preoperative stay	

Reprinted with permission from *AORN Journal*, Vol 49, p 508, February 1989.
Copyright © AORN Inc, 10170 East Mississippi Avenue, Denver, CO, 80231.

TABLE **12**
Drugs That Delay Wound Healing

Anticoagulants	Colchicine
Cause hematoma formation	Arrests cell replication
Anti-inflammatory agents	Suppresses collagen transport
Suppress inflammation	Diphenylhydantoin
Suppress protein synthesis	Causes hypertrophic scars
Suppress contraction	Methysergide
Suppress epithelialization	Causes excessive scarring
Chemotherapeutic agents	Penicillin
Arrest cell replication	Releases penicillamine
Suppress inflammation	Pentazocine
Suppress protein synthesis	May cause fibrosis

Adapted from Rothrock, J. C. (ed) (1987). *The RN first assistant: An expanded perioperative nursing role* (p. 199). Philadelphia: J. B. Lippincott.

TABLE **13**

Typical Appearance Times of Complications After Major Abdominal Surgery

Type of Complication	Postoperative Day									
	1	2	3	4	5	6	7	8	9	10
Pulmonary	X	X								
Ear, nose, and throat	X	X	X							
Urinary tract			X	X	X					
Thromboembolic						X	X	X	X	X	X
Wound infection, deep abscess					X	X	X	X	X	X	X
Anastomotic leaks and abscess							X	X	X		

Adapted from Polk, H. S., Stone, H. H., Gardener, B. (eds) (1987). *Basic surgery* (3rd ed). (p. 706). East Norwalk, Conn: Appleton-Century-Crofts.

INTERVENTIONS FOR WOUND INFECTIONS
- Assess the wound for cellulitis, phlegmon, or lymphangitis.
- Look for systemic infection.
- Determine the patient's comfort level and assess the skin condition.
- Assess the wound for gas formation (most common sites are the extremities after traumatic injury).

TABLE **14**

Postoperative Wound Infections

Onset (Postoperative Day)	Usual Pathogen
1–3	Clostridium perfringens and related species
2–3	Streptococcus
3–5	Staphylococcus
>5	Gram-negative rod
>5	Symbiotic

From Polk, H. S., Stone, H. H., Gardener, B. (eds) (1987). *Basic surgery* (3rd ed). (p. 151). East Norwalk, Conn: Appleton-Century-Crofts.

- Monitor the white blood cell count.
- Culture the wound if necessary.
- Refer for medical treatment if indicated.
- In the event of infection, implement measures to reduce pain, such as elevating the affected area to decrease edema and applying moist heat for patient comfort.
- Administer antibiotics as ordered.
- If antibiotics have not been ordered, recommend an appropriate antibiotic to the physician.
- Implement patient education measures regarding the status of infection and its treatment.
- Reevaluate the affected area after 24 hours of antibiotic therapy.
- Document findings and activities according to institutional policy.

Wound Abscess
- The abscessed area is usually tender to the touch.
- When touched in the abscess area, the patient most likely indicates pain.
- The patient may be febrile.
- Taut skin and tissue necrosis further confirm the presence of an abscess.

Wound Appearance	Other Signs
Brawny, hemorrhagic, cool, occasional gaseous crepitation, putrid dishwater exudate, intense local pain	High sustained fever (39–40°C), irrational, leukocytosis >15,000/mm³, occasional jaundice
Erythematous, warm, tender, occasionally hemorrhagic with blebs, serous exudate	High spiking fever (up to 39–40°C), irrational at times, leukocytosis >15,000/mm³, rare jaundice
Erythematous, warm, tender, purulent exudate	High spiking fever (up to 38–39°C), irrational at times, leukocytosis 12,000–20,000/mm³, rare jaundice
Erythematous, warm, tender, purulent exudate	Sustained low-grade to moderate fever (38–39°C), rational, leukocytosis 10,000–16,000/mm³
Erythematous, warm, tender, focal necrosis, purulent, putrid exudate	Moderate to high fever (38–40°C), mentation variable, leukocytosis >15,000/mm³, occasional jaundice

INTERVENTIONS FOR WOUND ABSCESS
- Assess the patient for signs of abscess.
- Look for systemic signs of infection.
- Determine the patient's comfort level.
- Assess the skin condition.
- Monitor the white blood cell count.
- Culture the wound if necessary.
- Refer for medical treatment if indicated.
- Implement measures to reduce pain as described for infection.
- Administer antibiotics as ordered.
- Implement wound care measures after the abscess has been drained.
- When repacking the wound, loosely pack it with material moistened in normal saline solution.
- Initiate measures to protect the skin from irritating drainage, tape, or chemicals.
- Daily assess the skin around the drainage site for signs of irritation or breakdown.
- Counsel the patient about her or his abscess, the planned treatment, and the probable clinical course.
- Show the patient how to care for the wound.
- Document findings and activities according to institutional policy.

Seroma

- Common in obese patients and in wounds with areas of undermined skin flaps.
- Consists of blood and protein-rich fluid.
- Seromas are sterile in the beginning but are susceptible to infections.
- The local swelling associated with a seroma may make the patient uncomfortable.
- The skin over and surrounding a seroma is usually not inflamed or compromised (Polk et al., 1987).

INTERVENTIONS FOR SEROMAS
- Assess the wound for signs of a seroma.
- Determine the patient's comfort level.
- Assess the skin condition.
- Monitor the white blood cell count.
- Culture the wound if necessary.
- Refer for medical treatment if indicated.
- Implement measures to reduce pain.
- Administer pain medication as ordered.
- Aspirate the seroma.
   1. Collect the supplies necessary to aspirate the seroma:

a. 20 to 35 ml syringe
b. 16- or 18-gauge needle
c. Skin-preparation solution
d. Adhesive bandage (Band-Aid)
e. 0.5 ml local anesthetic (optional)
f. 3 ml syringe
g. 25-gauge needle

2. Prepare the skin with alcohol or an antiseptic of preference.
3. After anesthetizing the skin with 0.5 ml of local anesthetic, insert the large-gauge needle attached to the large syringe and evacuate fluid until the cavity has collapsed.
4. After withdrawing the needle, cover the site with an adhesive bandage to keep fluid from leaking from the needle wound.

- Assist in inserting a suction wound drainage device.
  1. Collect the supplies necessary to insert the suction wound drainage device:
     a. Skin-preparation solution
     b. Wound-drainage device of choice
     c. Four drape towels
     d. No. 15 or 11 blade and No. 3 knife handle
     e. Hemostat
     f. Needle holder
     g. Suture scissors
     h. 10 ml syringe
     i. 18- and 25-gauge needles
     j. 10 to 20 ml of local anesthetic agent
     k. Dressing sponges
     l. Tape
     m. Sterile gloves
  2. Prepare the skin with alcohol or an antiseptic of preference.
  3. Don sterile gloves and prepare supplies.
  4. Draw up local anesthetic agent with an 18-gauge needle.
  5. Cut the drain to the proper length and attach it to the reservoir.
  6. Square off the area with sterile drapes.
  7. Numb the skin and track site to the seroma with the 25-gauge needle and a local anesthetic agent.
  8. Make an incision approximately 2 cm in length well below the seroma site. With a hemostat, make a track through the subcutaneous layer to the seroma. Fluid may leak out at this point.
  9. Insert the drain through the track into the seroma cavity with a hemostat.
  10. Close the incision and secure the tubing with suture. Dress the wound. Reassess the wound daily and check the amount of drainage.

- Counsel the patient about the seroma, the treatment, and the probable clinical course.
- Teach the patient how to care for the wound.
- Document findings and activities according to institutional policy.

Gas Gangrene

- Sudden onset
- High fever
- Intense local pain
- Incredibly foul odor
- Crepitant, dark, and cool tissue
- Sometimes hemorrhagic areas at the margin of the infection
- Possible signs of jaundice, confusion, moribundity, tachycardia, and dyspnea

INTERVENTIONS FOR GAS GANGRENE

- Assess the wound for signs of gas gangrene.
- Check for signs of systemic infection.
- Assess the patient's comfort level.
- Assess the patient's skin.
- Check the wound for crepitus.
- Assess the mental status.
- Check the white blood cell count.
- Culture the wound if necessary.
- Refer for medical treatment as indicated.
- Implement measures to reduce pain.
- Implement safety measures if the patient is confused.
- Administer antibiotics as ordered.
- If antibiotics have not been ordered, recommend an appropriate antibiotic to the physician.
- Counsel the patient about the infection, the treatment plan, and the probable clinical course.
- Show the patient how to care for the wound.
- Follow institutional policies regarding the isolation of patients with gas gangrene.
- Assist with the surgical débridement of the wound.
- Document findings and activities according to institutional policy.

Wound Dehiscence and Evisceration

- If wound dehiscence happens, it will usually occur about the fifth postoperative day.
- Infection is the precipitating factor in 50% of cases.
- Wound edge ischemia and wound closure under extreme tension are other usual causes of wound dehiscence.
- Before dehiscence occurs, the patient has serosanguineous drainage.

- After the wound begins to separate, evisceration may occur.
- The patient often reports that "something gave way." The treatment of wound dehiscence or evisceration is surgical closure.

INTERVENTIONS FOR WOUND DEHISCENCE AND EVISCERATION

- During the first 5 to 6 days of convalescence, check the wound for signs of impending separation.
- Look for serosanguineous drainage.
- Assess the patient's level of comfort.
- Refer for medical treatment immediately in case of dehiscence or evisceration.
- If evisceration occurs, implement measures to ensure patient safety.
  1. Place the patient in a supine position.
  2. Cover the wound with sterile towels moistened with saline solution.
  3. Implement measures to prevent hypovolemic shock.
  4. Prepare the patient for surgical closure of the wound.
- Counsel the patient about the wound, the treatment plan, and the probable clinical course.
- Assist with surgical closure of the wound.
- Document findings and activities according to institutional policy.

Nonhealing Wounds (Table 15)

INTERVENTIONS FOR NONHEALING WOUNDS

- Assess the wound for signs of nonhealing.
- Review preoperatively and postoperatively the patient's history for risk factors.

TABLE **15**
Causes of Nonhealing Wounds

Cancer	Infections
Basal cell carcinoma	Inadequate nutrition
Leukemia	Starvation (protein depletion)
Melanoma	Inflammatory bowel disease
Squamous cell carcinoma	(malabsorption syndromes)
Chronic trauma	Radiation
Factitious ulcer	Locally irradiated tissues
Hyperactivity	Radiation enteritis
Peripheral neuropathy	Vascular disorders
Poor hygiene	Arterial ischemia and atherosclerosis
Proximal nerve injury	Diabetes
Pruritus	Decubital ulcers
Drug therapy	Arteritis

Adapted from Rothrock, J. C. (ed) (1987). *The RN first assistant: An expanded perioperative nursing role* (p. 194). Philadelphia: J. B. Lippincott.

- Assess the white blood cell count.
- Culture the wound if necessary.
- Refer for medical treatment if indicated.
- Implement measures to reduce discomfort, if present.
- Implement measures to eliminate infection, hematomas, seromas, and retained foreign substances.
- Do not use cytotoxic substances and chemicals to clean the wound. Use normal saline.
- Counsel the patient about the wound, the treatment plan, and the probable clinical course.
- Show the patient how to care for the wound.
- Document findings and activities according to institutional policy.

Recognizing Fever, Tachycardia, Pulmonary Complications, Thrombophlebitis, Urinary Tract Infections, and Adynamic Ileus

Fever

- Can occur at any time postoperatively.
- Transient low-grade postoperative fever is considered normal.
- Fever may be present after blood transfusion.
- If inflamed tissue was removed during surgery, expect a constantly elevated temperature 3 to 5 days postoperatively.
- A spiking temperature, one that is intermittently high, may mean a more serious problem, such as bacterial seeding into the bloodstream.
- Spiking temperatures during the first 2 days postoperatively are usually pulmonary in origin.
- From the fourth to the seventh day, suspect wound complications.
- Fevers on the sixth to the ninth days are commonly attributable to intra-abdominal abscesses or anastomotic leaks.
- Thrombophlebitis can cause a fever from the sixth to the tenth day.

INTERVENTIONS FOR FEVER

- Evaluate the fever pattern and assess for the underlying cause.
- Refer for medical treatment when indicated.
- Implement measures to educate the patient regarding the elevated temperature, the treatment, and the probable clinical course.
- Document findings and activities according to institutional policy.

Tachycardia

- Related to fever; lack of a medication routinely taken by the patient, such as digitalis; relative hypotension (for example, if the patient is ordinarily hypertensive); inadequate pain relief; and apprehension.

- Treatment depends on the underlying cause.

INTERVENTIONS FOR TACHYCARDIA

- Assess the patient for the underlying cause.
- Refer for medical treatment if indicated.
- Implement measures to educate the patient regarding tachycardia, the treatment, and the probable clinical course.
- Document findings and activities according to institutional policy.

Pulmonary Complications

- Pulmonary complications usually appear during the first 2 days postoperatively.
- Involve atelectasis, infiltrate, or effusions
- Accompanied by an elevated temperature, tachycardia, restlessness, elevated white blood cell count, lowered partial pressure of oxygen, increased partial pressure of carbon dioxide, dyspnea, increased respiratory rate, pallor, and shortness of breath.
- In severe cases, hypoxia can cause deterioration of mental status and level of consciousness and cyanosis.
- If the patient does not cough effectively, portions of the bronchial tree can become plugged with mucus.
- Pain and splinting are major causes of ineffective cough.
- Adequate pain relief can assist the patient to move the secretions; however, narcotics can depress respiratory effort.
- Segmental atelectasis can occur with bed rest or inadequate intraoperative ventilation.
- Treatment modalities for pulmonary complications
  1. Increase in activity, such as ambulation
  2. Incentive spirometer
  3. Postural drainage
  4. Percussion
  5. Inspiration of humidified air
  6. Intermittent positive-pressure breathing treatments with mucolytic agents
  7. Tracheal suction
  8. Adequate fluid intake

PNEUMONIA

- If conditions persist, look for signs of pneumonia
  1. Infiltrate x-ray films
  2. Diminished breath signs (especially in the lower lobes)
  3. Crackles
  4. Positive sputum cultures, especially for massive or subtle aspiration

POSTOPERATIVE PLEURAL EFFUSIONS

- Can be caused by pneumonia, pulmonary embolus, congestive heart failure, or subdiaphragmatic abscess.
- The most common cause of pleural effusion is pneumonia (see above).
- Plural effusions
  1. Are often visible on chest x-ray films
  2. Tend to muffle all sounds when auscultated
  3. Have percussion notes that are dull
  4. Result in decrease in or absence of breath sounds

PULMONARY EMBOLUS

- Look for sudden chest or shoulder pain, dyspnea, tachycardia, hypotension, pallor, cyanosis, restlessness, and hypoxia.
- Look for significant and sudden falls in pulse oximeter readings
- Oxygen pressure is significantly lower, even reaching dangerous levels.
- Sudden death can occur.
- Immediate resuscitative intervention may be required.
- If suspected, obtain order for peripheral venograms, pulmonary arteriograms, and lung scans for confirmation.
- Surgeon my order anticoagulants such as a continuous heparin infusion or intermittent heparin injections.
- Long-term oral anticoagulant therapy may be desirable.
- Preventive measures include prevention of thrombophlebitis.

CONGESTIVE HEART FAILURE

- Postoperative fluid overload can lead to congestive heart failure.
- Congestive heart failure is characterized by vascular congestion and the inability of the heart to pump enough blood to meet the body's metabolic needs.
- It is essential to monitor patient's intake and output and daily weights (especially for patients with preexisting congestive heart failure).
- It may be difficult to differentiate between overhydration and third spacing of fluids.
- Central venous pressure monitoring is inadequate for this complication. Monitoring pulmonary wedge pressures with a Swan-Ganz catheter is more appropriate.
- Diuretics and inotropic drugs may be used in the treatment of overhydration.

SUBDIAPHRAGMATIC ABSCESSES

- Subdiaphragmatic abscesses irritate the diaphragm and may create a pleural effusion.
- Look for pain on light palpation of the subcostal margin of the affected side.
- Abscesses produce a dull sound when percussed.

- Look for gradually deteriorating arterial blood gas measurements and pulse oximeter readings.
- Abscesses are readily seen with sonography or computed tomography.
- The treatment
    1. Surgical or percutaneous drainage of the abscess
    2. Effusion may be aspirated
    3. If the effusion is severe enough, the surgeon may choose to insert a chest tube to drain the effusion

INTERVENTIONS FOR PULMONARY COMPLICATIONS

- Assess pulmonary complications.
- Assess the patient's activity level and ability to ambulate.
- Monitor arterial blood gas values and pulse oximeter readings.
- Evaluate the effectiveness of the cough.
- Evaluate the use of respiration-depressing drugs.
- Monitor intake and output.
- Monitor pulmonary wedge pressures.
- Refer for medical treatment, if indicated, or immediately in the event of a pulmonary embolus.
- In the event of pulmonary complications, recommend appropriate diagnostic and/or treatment modalities.
- Assess the effectiveness of measures to prevent pulmonary infiltrates and pneumonia.
- Assess the effectiveness of measures to prevent pulmonary embolus.
- Implement measures to educate the patient regarding her or his role in preventing pulmonary complications.
- If complications occur, educate the patient regarding the treatment and the probable clinical course.
- Document findings and activities according to institutional policy.

Thrombophlebitis

- Thrombophlebitis results from inactivity with venous stasis in the lower extremities or as a complication of intravenous catheters.
- Prolonged venous cannulation or chemical reaction from intravenous medications can cause a peripheral vein to thrombose.
- The most serious form of thrombophlebitis occurs in the deep veins of the legs. This can be precipitated by pelvic edema resulting from surgical procedures (e.g., hysterectomy and hip procedures), intraoperative positioning that restricts venous return, or postoperative bed rest.
- If a clot embolizes to the pulmonary circulation, sudden death can occur.

- Assess the patient for pain, local tenderness, swelling in the calf and foot, and transient fever.
- Palpate for deep thrombophlebitis.
  1. With the patient's leg flexed at the knee and relaxed, press the calf muscles against the tibia with the fingertips.
  2. Feel for increased firmness or muscle tension.
- Prevent thrombophlebitis by maintaining high venous flow.
  1. Apply elastic stockings.
  2. Elevate the patient's legs.
  3. Encourage muscular exercise.
- Instruct the patient to avoid having the legs in a dependent position unless he or she is ambulating.
- The physician may prescribe continuous heparin infusions or intermittent heparin injections.

INTERVENTIONS FOR THROMBOPHLEBITIS

- Assess for venous thrombosis.
- Implement measures for patient comfort.
- Encourage early ambulation.
- Implement measures to educate the patient regarding his or her role in preventing thrombophlebitis.
- If complications occur, perform the following:
  1. Refer for medical treatment.
  2. Educate the patient regarding treatment and the probable clinical course.
  3. Assess the effectiveness of measures to treat thrombophlebitis.
- Document findings and activities according to institutional policy.

Urinary Tract Infections

- Urinary tract infections can be diagnosed from the patient's description of the problem.
- Patients may express an urgent and frequent need to evacuate small amounts of urine. They may also verbalize bladder fullness, burning on urination, and suprapubic distention. Urine may be foul-smelling or cloudy.
- The patient may have chills and fever. Urinalysis shows many white blood cells in the urine.
- A culture produces bacteria.
- Infections can be treated with the administration of sulfa drugs or antibiotics if necessary.
- Absence of urination with suprapubic distention means urinary retention.
- Measures to prevent urinary retention are activities that facilitate voiding, such as running water, helping male patients stand to void, and offering a bedpan or assistance to the bathroom every 2 to 3 hours.

- If these measures prove inadequate, a catheter should be inserted intermittently or an indwelling catheter may be used.

INTERVENTIONS FOR URINARY TRACT INFECTIONS

- Assess for signs of urinary tract infection.
- In the event of urinary tract infection, perform the following:
  1. Refer for medical treatment.
  2. Implement measures for patient comfort.
  3. Educate the patient regarding treatment and the probable clinical course.
  4. Assess the effectiveness of measures to treat urinary tract infection.
- Document findings and activities according to institutional policy.

Adynamic Ileus

- Adynamic ileus is a common occurrence after abdominal surgery.
- The bowel remains flaccid for several days.
- Intestinal motility is ineffective in moving contents along the tract, or it stops entirely.
- Adynamic ileus is frequently associated with thoracic, retroperitoneal, and abdominal trauma, as well as spinal cord injuries.
- Less frequent causes are metabolic and vascular.
- Low serum potassium levels paralyze the smooth muscle of the bowel.
- Surgical intervention with resection of the ischemic bowel and restoration of the blood supply is urgent.
- Adynamic ileus, unaccompanied by mesenteric vascular insufficiency or peritonitis, exhibits diminished to absent bowel sounds, abdominal distention, nontender abdomen, nausea, vomiting, and signs of extracellular fluid loss.
- Generally, the patient is not concerned about the abdomen because it is not tender. The patient may express "feeling full."
- Postoperative ileus in the absence of metabolic or vascular insufficiencies is a self-limiting condition.
- The treatment of adynamic ileus is to withhold oral intake until bowel function returns.
- The patient may be relieved by the insertion of a nasogastric tube to evacuate the stomach contents.
- The first sign of returning bowel function is the presence of active sounds or the passage of flatus. If adynamic ileus is persistent, the RNFA may suspect peritonitis, potassium depletion, or wound dehiscence.

INTERVENTIONS FOR ADYNAMIC ILEUS

- Assess the patient for signs of prolonged ileus.
- Assess the comfort level.

- In the event of prolonged adynamic ileus, perform the following:
  1. Refer for medical treatment.
  2. Implement measures for patient comfort.
  3. Implement measures to educate the patient regarding the reasons for ileus and when bowel function is expected to return.
- Document findings and activities according to institutional policy.

Assessing Postoperative Comfort Level

- Postoperative pain, nausea, and vomiting are the most common causes of alteration in comfort.
- The assessment of pain is an ongoing process that often begins as the patient returns to consciousness in the PACU. Figure 1

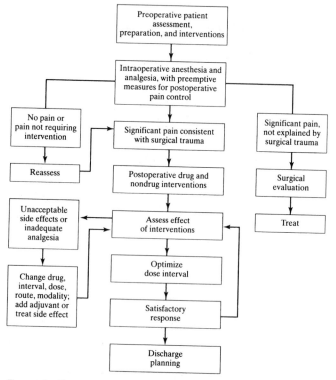

FIGURE 1 Flow chart depicting postoperative pain management. (Adapted from *Acute pain management in adults: Operative procedures. Quick reference guide for clinicians.* AHCPR Pub No. 92-0019. [1992]. [p. 4]. Rockville, Md: Agency for Health Care Policy and Research, Public Health Service, U.S. Department of Health and Human Services.)

presents a flow chart for the management of postoperative pain.
- Pain is a subjective experience. Use of a pain-intensity scale to assess the patient's pain is very helpful (Fig. 2).
- Figure 3 illustrates the potential detrimental effects of pain on the patient.

Signs and Symptoms of Pain (Kim and Moritz, 1982)
- Guarding or protective behavior
- Self-focusing
- Altered time perception
- Withdrawal from social contact

Simple Descriptive Pain Intensity Scale[1]

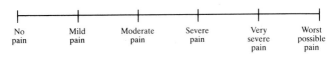

0–10 Numeric Pain Intensity Scale[1]

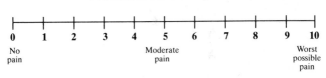

Visual Analog Scale (VAS)[2]

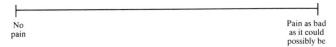

FIGURE 2 Examples of pain intensity scales. [1]If used as a graphic rating scale, a 10 cm baseline is recommended. [2]A 10 cm baseline is recommended for VAS scales. (Adapted from *Acute pain management in adults: Operative procedures. Quick reference guide for clinicians.* AHCPR Pub No. 92-0019. [1992]. [p. 14]. Rockville, Md: Agency for Health Care Policy and Research, Public Health Service, U.S. Department of Health and Human Services.)

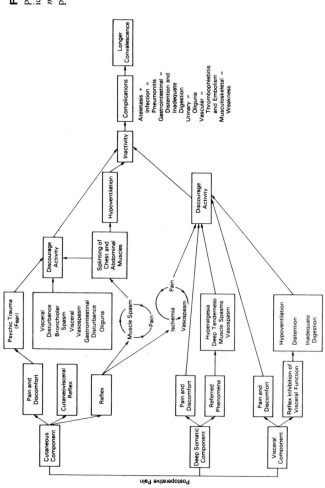

FIGURE 3 Possible effects of postoperative pain. (From Bonica, J. J. [1953]. *The management of pain* [p. 1241]. Philadelphia: Lea & Febiger.)

298

- Impaired thought processes
- Distraction behavior
- Crying
- Moaning
- Restlessness
- Facial mask of pain
- Eyes dull
- Fixed or scattered movement
- Grimace
- Alteration in muscle tone (may be listless to rigid)
- Autonomic responses not seen in stable chronic pain
- Diaphoresis
- Blood pressure and pulse rate change
- Pupillary dilation
- Increased or decreased respiratory rate

Recommended Dose and Effects of Medication Given to Control or Relieve Pain (Tables 16 and 17)

Scientific Evidence for Interventions to Manage Pain in Adults (Table 18)

INTERVENTIONS
- Assess the patient for level of pain relief (see Fig. 2).
- Assess how the patient responds to pain.
- In the event of inadequately controlled postoperative pain, perform the following:
  1. Refer for medical treatment if indicated.
  2. Implement measures to educate the patient regarding his or her role in pain control.
  3. Implement nonpharmacologic measures for pain relief.
- Document findings and activities according to institutional policy.

Assessing Nausea and Vomiting

- Narcotic-induced nausea and vomiting usually occur shortly after the medication has been administered.
- The patient may state that she or he thinks the pain medicine is making her or him sick.
- The treatment is to administer an antiemetic and change the type of or eliminate the narcotic.
- A nasogastric tube is rarely necessary for narcotic-induced nausea and vomiting.

INTERVENTIONS
- Assess the patient for the causes of nausea and vomiting.
- Refer for medical treatment if indicated.
- Document findings and activities according to institutional policy.

TABLE 16

Dosing Data for Nonsteroidal Anti-inflammatory Drugs (NSAIDs)

Drug	Usual Adult Dose
Oral NSAIDs	
Acetaminophen	650–975 mg q4h
Aspirin	650–975 mg q4h
Choline magnesium trisalicylate (Trislisate)	1000–1500 mg bid
Diflunisal (Dolobid)	1000 mg initial dose followed by 500 mg q12h
Etodolac (Lodine)	200–400 mg q6–8h
Fenoprofen calcium (Nalfon)	200 mg q4–6h
Ibuprofen (Motrin, others)	400 mg q4–6h
Ketoprofen (orudis)	25–75 mg q6–8h
Magnesium salicylate	650 mg q4h
Meclofenamate sodium (Meclomen)	50 mg q4–6h
Mefenamic acid (Ponstel)	250 mg q6h
Naproxen (Naprosyn)	500 mg initial dose followed by 250 mg q6–8h
Naproxen sodium (Anaprox)	550 mg initial dose followed by 275 mg q6–8h
Salsalate (Disalcid, others)	500 mg q4h
Sodium salicylate	325–650 mg q3–4h
Parenteral NSAID	
Ketorolac tromethamine (Toradol)	30 or 60 mg IM initial dose followed by 15 or 30 mg q6h; oral dose following IM dosage: 10 mg q6–8h

Note: Only the above NSAIDs have FDA approval for use as simple analgesics, but clinical experience has been gained with other drugs as well.

*Drug recommendations are limited to NSAIDs where pediatric dosing experience is available.

†Contraindicated in presence of fever or other evidence of viral illness.

Adapted from *Acute pain management in adults: Operative procedures. Quick reference guide for clinicians.* AHCPR Pub No. 92–0019. (1992). (pp. 18–19). Rockville, Md: Agency for Health Care Policy and Research, Public Health Service, U.S. Department of Health and Human Services.

Ensuring the Proper Functioning of Devices to Assist Recovery

- Several devices are commonly used to assist the patient in recovering from surgical intervention. These include nasogastric tubes, dressings, chest tubes, closed drainage systems, and open drains.

Usual Pediatric Dose*	Comments
10–15 mg/kg q4h	Acetaminophen lacks the peripheral anti-inflammatory activity of other NSAIDs
10–15 mg/kg q4h†	The standard against which other NSAIDs are compared. Inhibits platelet aggregation; may cause postoperative bleeding
25 mg/kg bid	May have minimal antiplatelet activity; also available as oral liquid
10 mg/kg q6–8h	Available as several brand names and as generic; also available as oral suspension
	Many brands and generic forms available
5 mg/kg q12h	Also available as oral liquid
	May have minimal antiplatelet activity
	Available in generic form from several distributors
	Intramuscular dose not to exceed 5 days

Nasogastric tubes

- The purpose of a nasogastric tube is to keep the stomach evacuated.
- Use to treat nausea and vomiting with distention from ileus.
- Restrict patient to nothing by mouth; therefore, the output should be made up almost entirely of gastric secretions.

TABLE 17

Dosing Data for Opioid Analgesics

Drug	Approximate Equianalgesic Dose	
	Oral	Parenteral
Opioid Agonist		
Morphine*	30 mg q3–4h (around-the-clock dosing)	10 mg q3–4h
	60 mg q3–4h (single dose or intermittent dosing)	
Codeine†	130 mg q3–4h	75 mg q3–4h
Hydromorphone* (Dilaudid)	7.5 mg q3–4h	1.5 mg q3–4h
Hydrocodone (in Lorcet, Lortab, Vicodin, others)	30 mg q3–4h	Not available
Levorphanol (Levo-Dromoran)	4 mg q6–8h	2 mg q6–8h
Meperidine (Demerol)	300 mg q2–3h	100 mg q3h
Methadone (Dolophine, others)	20 mg q6–8h	10 mg q6–8h
Oxycodone (Roxicodone, also in Percocet, Percodan, Tylox, others)	30 mg q3–4h	Not available
Oxymorphone† (Numorphan)	Not available	1 mg q3–4h
Opioid Agonist-Antagonist and Partial Agonist		
Buprenorphine (Buprenex)	Not available	0.3–0.4 mg q6–8h
Butorphanol (Stadol)	Not available	2 mg q3–4h
Nalbuphine (Nubain)	Not available	10 mg q3–4h
Pentazocine (Talwin, others)	150 mg q3–4h	60 mg q3–4h

Note: Published tables vary in the suggested doses that are equianalgesic to morphine. Clinical response is the criterion that must be applied for each patient; titration to clinical response is necessary. Because there is not complete cross tolerance among these drugs, it is usually necessary to use a lower than equianalgesic dose when changing drugs and to retitrate to response.
Caution: Recommended doses do not apply to patients with renal or hepatic insufficiency or other conditions affecting drug metabolism and kinetics.
*For morphine, hydromorphone, and oxymorphone, rectal administration is an alternate route for patients unable to take oral medications, but equianalgesic doses may differ from oral and parenteral doses because of pharmacokinetic differences.
†Caution: Codeine doses above 65 mg often are not appropriate because of diminishing incremental analgesia with increasing doses but continually increasing constipation and other side effects.

- Normally, the stomach secretes up to 500 to 1000 ml/day. After the nasogastric tube output has dropped below this level, the tube is no longer therapeutic and should be removed.
- Severe ear pain can mean acute otitis media if the nasogastric tube occludes the eustachian tube. The nasogastric tube should be removed immediately. It may be repositioned to the other nostril if necessary.

Dressings

- The purpose of dressings is to provide a clean environment for the incision, thus preventing the introduction of pathogens into the wound before the wound edges can seal.
- Dressings also wick drainage up and away from the skin.
- Other functions are to provide pressure, hemostasis, support to the wound, or débridement of the wound (Fay, 1987).

Recommended Starting Dose (adults more than 50 kg body weight)		Recommended Starting Dose (children and adults less than 50 kg body weight)‡	
Oral	Parenteral	Oral	Parenteral
30 mg q3–4h	10 mg q3–4h	0.3 mg/kg q3–4h	0.1 mg/kg q3–4h
60 mg q3–4h	60 mg q2h (intramuscular/ subcutaneous)	1 mg/kg q3–4h§	Not recommended
6 mg q3–4h	1.5 mg q3–4h	0.06 mg/kg q3–4h	0.015 mg/kg q3–4h
10 mg q3–4h	Not available	0.2 mg/kg q3–4h§	Not available
4 mg q6–8h	2 mg q6–8h	0.04 mg/kg q6–8h	0.02 mg/kg q6–8h
Not recommended	100 mg q3h	Not recommended	0.75 mg/kg q2–3h
20 mg q6–8h	10 mg q6–8h	0.2 mg/kg q6–8h	0.1 mg/kg q6–8h
10 mg q3–4h	Not available	0.2 mg/kg q3–4h§	Not available
Not available	1 mg q3–4h	Not recommended	Not recommended
Not available	0.4 mg q6–8h	Not available	0.004 mg/kg q6–8h
Not available	2 mg q3–4h	Not available	Not recommended
Not available	10 mg q3–4h	Not available	0.1 mg/kg q3–4h
50 mg q4–6h	Not recommended	Not recommended	Not recommended

‡Caution: Doses listed for patients with body weight less than 50 cannot be used as initial starting doses in babies less than 6 months of age. Consult the *Clinical practice guideline for acute pain management: Operative or medical procedures and trauma* section on management of pain in neonates for recommendations.

§Caution: Doses of aspirin and acetaminophen in combination opioid/NSAID preparations must also be adjusted to the patient's body weight.

Adapted from *Acute pain management in adults: Operative procedures. Quick reference guide for clinicians.* AHCPR Pub No. 92–0019. (1992). (pp. 20–21). Rockville, Md: Agency for Health Care Policy and Research, Public Health Service, U.S. Department of Health and Human Services.

- Pressure dressings may offer some benefit in reducing edema; however, the risk of tape burns of the skin is high.
- Dressings for hemostasis are inappropriate. The control of bleeding is best achieved intraoperatively.
- Pressure dressings should be limited to immobilizing and supporting the wound. One appropriate use of the pressure dressing is on skin grafts.
- Pressure ensures that the donor skin stays in contact with the blood supply at the graft site.
- Wounds may be débrided by the frequent changing of dressing materials loosely packed into an open wound.

Chest Tubes

- The purpose of chest tubes is to evacuate air, fluid, or pus from the pleural space so that the lung can inflate completely.

TABLE **18**
Scientific Evidence for Interventions to Manage Pain in Adults

Intervention*	Type of Evidence
Pharmacologic Interventions	
NSAIDs	
Oral (alone)	Ib, IV
Oral (adjunct to opioid)	Ia, IV
Parenteral (ketorolac)	Ib, IV
Opioids	
Oral	IV
Intramuscular	Ib, IV
Subcutaneous	Ib, IV
Intravenous	Ib, IV
PCA (systemic)	Ia, IV
Epidural and intrathecal	Ia, IV
Local Anesthetics	
Epidural and intrathecal	Ia, IV
Peripheral nerve block	Ia, IV
Nonpharmacologic Interventions	
Simple Relaxation (begin preoperatively)	
Jaw relaxation	Ia, IIa, IIb, IV
Progressive muscle relaxation	
Simple imagery	
Music	Ib, IIa, IV
Complex Relaxation (begin preoperatively)	
Biofeedback	Ib, IIa, IV
Imagery	Ib, IIa, IIb, IV
Education/Instruction (begin preoperatively)	Ia, IIa, IIb, IV
Transcutaneous Electrical Nerve Stimulation	Ia, IIa, III, IV

*Insufficient scientific evidence is available to provide specific recommendations regarding the use of hypnosis, acupuncture, and other physical modalities for relief of postoperative pain.

Type of Evidence—Key

Ia, Evidence obtained from meta-analysis of randomized controlled trials; Ib, Evidence obtained from at least one randomized controlled trial; IIa, Evidence obtained from at least one well-designed controlled study without randomization; IIb, Evidence obtained from at least one other type of well-designed quasi-experimental study; III, Evidence obtained from well-designed nonexperimental descriptive studies, such as comparative studies, correlational studies, and case studies; IV, Evidence obtained from expert committee reports or opinions and/or clinical experiences of respected authorities.

Effective for mild to moderate pain. Begin preoperatively. Relatively contraindicated in patients with renal disease and risk of or actual coagulopathy. May mask fever.

Poteniating effect resulting in opioid sparing. Begin preoperatively. Cautions as above.

Effective for moderate to severe pain. Expensive. Useful where opioids are contraindicated, especially to avoid respiratory depression and sedation. Advance to opioid.

As effective as parenteral in appropriate doses. Use as soon as oral medication is tolerated. Route of choice.

Has been the standard parenteral route, but injections painful and absorption unreliable. Hence, avoid this route when possible.

Preferable to intramuscular for low-volume continuous infusion. Injections painful and absorption unreliable. Avoid this route for long-term repetitive dosing.

Parenteral route of choice after major surgery. Suitable for titrated bolus or continuous administration (including PCA), but requires monitoring. Significant risk of respiratory depression with inappropriate dosing.

Intravenous or subcutaneous routes recommended. Good, steady level of analgesia. Popular with patients but requires special infusion pumps and staff education. See cautions about opioids above.

When suitable, provides good analgesia. Significant risk of respiratory depression, sometimes delayed in onset. Requires careful monitoring. Use of infusion pumps requires additional equipment and staff education.

Limited indications. Expensive if infusion pumps are employed. Effective regional analgesia. Opioid sparing. Addition of opioid to local anesthetic may improve analgesia. Risks of hypotension, weakness, numbness. Use of infusion pump requires additional equipment and staff.

Limited indications and duration of action. Effective regional analgesia. Opioid sparing.

Effective in reducing mild to moderate pain and as an adjunct to analgesic drugs for severe pain. Use when patients express an interest in relaxation. Requires 3–5 min of staff time for instruction.

Both patient-preferred and "easy listening" music are effective in reducing mild to moderate pain.

Effective in reducing mild to moderate pain and operative site muscle tension. Requires skilled personnel and special equipment.

Effective for reduction of mild to moderate pain. Requires skilled personnel.

Effective for reduction of pain. should include sensory and procedural information and instruction aimed at reducing activity-related pain. Requires 5–15 min of staff time.

Effective in reducing pain and improving physical function. Requires skilled personnel and special equipment. May be useful as an adjunct to drug therapy.

Note: References are available in the *Guideline report. Acute pain management: Operative or medical procedures and trauma.* AHCPR Pub No. 92–0001. Rockville, Md: Agency for Health Care Policy and Research, Public Health Service, U.S. Department of Health and Human Services. In press.

Adapted from *Acute pain management in adults: Operative procedures. Quick reference guide for clinicians.* AHCPR Pub No. 92–0019. (1992). (pp. 16–17). Rockville, Md: Agency for Health Care Policy and Research, Public Health Service, U.S. Department of Health and Human Services.

- Chest tubes are inserted intraoperatively after thoracic procedures.
- Chest tubes may be used in cases of spontaneous pneumothorax, which can occur while the patient is being mechanically ventilated.
- Iatrogenic pneumothorax (penetration of the pleural space with a needle during insertion of a subclavian catheter) is also treated with chest tubes.
- Pleural effusions (causes discussed above) are drained through chest tubes.
- If the skin at the insertion site is not well closed, air may be pulled into the chest around it. A reliable method to prevent this is to place three sutures intraoperatively. The first two close the incision around the tube and secure the tube in place. The third suture is placed so that it can be tied to close the skin when the chest tube is removed. A frequently used, but less reliable, method to make the seal around the tube airtight is to apply petroleum jelly (Vaseline)–impregnated gauze at the insertion site. Pursestring sutures in the skin around the tube provide an airtight seal; however, they are likely to cause necrosis of the skin.
- The decision to remove the chest tube depends on its function. If its purpose is to drain fluid and superlative exudate, it may be removed when less than 200 ml/day is draining from the chest. If the purpose is to evacuate air, it may be removed when there is no evidence of an air leak. An air leak is present if, when the patient coughs, air bubbles appear in the water seal of the system.

Closed Drains

- Closed drains are placed to evacuate fluid that may accumulate or that has already accumulated in a wound.
- They are used more often in nonsuppurative wounds than in suppurative wounds.
- They are composed of a collection unit, extension tubing, and drainage tubing. Drainage tubing is available in a variety of sizes and styles. Most rely on some form of vacuum to facilitate the evacuation of fluid.
- These may be pumping devices that are stationary (wall suction with regulator), a line-powered pump (Gomco), or a manually activated device. Vacuum pressure is fixed for manually controlled systems, whereas it can be regulated with stationary or line-powered devices.
- The most common reasons for failure of closed drainage systems are inadequate tube diameter, improper placement or displacement of tube, loss of vacuum pressure, occlusion of the drain fenestration with clot or tissue, and retrograde contamination of the wound during emptying (Fay, 1987).

Open Drains
- Open drains are used for the same reasons as closed systems.
- They are used more in suppurative than in nonsuppurative wounds.
- They ensure that the wound stays open for the drainage of thick suppurative and necrotic materials.
- They are made of soft latex or rigid plastic or Silastic tubing in a variety of styles, sizes, and lengths.
- Open drains are secured with a safety pin or sutured to the skin. This prevents the drain from becoming dislodged and being pulled either into or out of the wound.
- A common practice with an open drain is to remove it gradually over several days. This allows the abscess cavity to drain and collapse as the drain is removed.
- The drainage can be irritating to the skin. Change dressing frequently and continuously assess the surrounding.
- Wound drainage bags protect the skin when there is a large amount of drainage.

Interventions
NASOGASTRIC TUBE
- Check proper functioning of the nasogastric tube.
- Check for proper positioning.
- Inject 10 to 20 ml of air and auscultate the stomach for the sound of air bubbles.
- Reposition if necessary.
- Note output.
- Check for patency.
- Irrigate with about 30 ml of saline solution.
- Check the suction unit.
- Place suction tubing in water.
- Assess the skin condition where the tube is secured.
- Assess the patient's comfort level.
- Implement measures to relieve dryness of mucous membranes.
- Remove the tube when its use is no longer therapeutic.
DRESSINGS
- Remove soiled dressings.
- Re-dress the wound only when drainage is present or if the purpose of the dressing is to débride the wound.
- Assess the skin condition under dressings and tape.
- Inspect wounds and the skin condition under splints and re-dress to continue support of the wound.
- Check that casts are intact.
CHEST TUBES
- Check the proper functioning of the system.
- Note whether the suction regulator is properly set.

- Note the amount and nature of the drainage.
- Ask the patient to cough.
- Note air bubbles in the water seal, which indicate that there is an air leak into the pleural space.
- Note whether air is being pulled into the chest at the insertion site.
- Assess the skin condition around the insertion site.
- Remove the tube when its use is no longer therapeutic.

REMOVAL OF CHEST TUBES

- Equipment and supplies
  1. Suture scissors
  2. Sterile gloves
  3. Sponges
  4. 2–0 or 3–0 silk suture on a cutting needle if a suture to tie has not been placed intraoperatively
- Optional supplies
  1. 3 ml syringe
  2. 2 to 3 ml of 1% lidocaine (Xylocaine)
  3. 25-gauge needle

PROCEDURE

- Open supplies.
- Don the gloves.
- Remove the dressing.
- Cut the sutures securing the tube to the skin.
- Ask the patient to inhale deeply and hold the breath.
- With a sponge and the fingertips, apply slight pressure to the skin above the insertion site as the tube is removed to prevent air from being pulled into the chest.
- Remove the tube in one steady motion.
- Apply firm pressure above the insertion site until the incision is closed.
- Tie the remaining suture to close the incision.
- Tell the patient that she or he may breathe normally.
- Inject local anesthetic, if indicated.
- Close with 2–0 or 3–0 silk on a cutting needle if no suture has been placed intraoperatively.
- Dress the wound.

CLOSED DRAINAGE SYSTEMS

- Check the proper functioning of the system.
- Check whether the vacuum is engaged.
- Note the amount of drainage collected in the past 24 hours.
- Compare daily amounts of drainage.
- Note the color, consistency, and odor of drainage.
- Check the patency of tubing.
- Ensure that the tubing is properly connected and free from kinks and that the system is airtight.

- Note the amount of drainage around the insertion site.
- Assess the skin condition at the insertion site.
- Remove when closed drainage is no longer therapeutic.

REMOVAL OF CLOSED DRAINAGE SYSTEMS

- Equipment and supplies
  1. Suture scissors
  2. Gloves
  3. Sponges
  4. Tape
- Procedure
  1. Open supplies.
  2. Don the gloves.
  3. Remove the dressing.
  4. Cut the suture securing the drain to the skin.
  5. Remove the drain in one steady motion.
  6. Dress the wound.

OPEN DRAINAGE SYSTEMS

- Note whether the drain is secured so that it does not come out or is not pulled into the wound.
- Check and compare the amount of drainage with that on previous days.
- Assess the color, consistency, and odor of drainage.
- Assess the skin condition around the insertion site.
- Gradually remove the drain.

REMOVAL OF OPEN DRAINAGE SYSTEMS

- Equipment and supplies
  1. Suture scissors
  2. Gloves
  3. Sponges
- Optional equipment and supplies
  1. Wound drainage bag or tape
  2. Safety pin or 4–0 nylon suture
  3. 3 ml syringe
  4. 2 to 3 ml of 1% lidocaine
  5. 25-gauge needle
- Procedure
  1. Open supplies.
  2. Don the gloves.
  3. Cut the suture, if any.
  4. Remove the drain about 5 cm.
  5. Reapply the safety pin, if applicable.
  6. Instill local anesthetic, if indicated.
  7. Suture the drain to the skin with nylon.
  8. Clean the skin around the wound.
  9. Apply the dressing or wound-drainage bag.
  10. Remove drain when its use is no longer therapeutic.

Bibliography

1992 Physicians' desk reference (46th ed). Montvale, NJ: Medical Economics Company.

A Job Analysis for the RN First Assistant. Denver: The National Certification Board: Perioperative Nursing, Inc.

Association for the Advancement of Medical Instrumentation. (1985, February). *Good hospital practice: Performance evaluation of ethylene oxide–ethylene oxide test packs.* Arlington, Va: The Association.

Association for the Advancement of Medical Instrumentation. (1981, March). *Good hospital practice: Ethylene oxide gas—Ventilation recommendations and safe use.* Arlington, Va: The Association.

Association for the Advancement of Medical Instrumentation. (1986, June). *Good hospital practice: Steam sterilization using the unwrapped method (flash sterilization).* Arlington, Va: The Association.

Association for the Advancement of Medical Instrumentation. (1980, January). *Good hospital practice: Steam sterilization and sterility assurance.* Arlington, Va: The Association.

Association of Operating Room Nurses. (1993). *Standards and recommended practices for perioperative nursing.* Denver: AORN.

Association of Operating Room Nurses. (1992). *Standards and recommended practices for perioperative nursing.* Denver: AORN.

Atkinson L. J., Kohn, M. L. (1986). *Berry and Kohn's introduction to operating room technique* (6th ed). New York: McGraw-Hill.

Ball, K. (1990). *Lasers: The perioperative challenge.* St. Louis: C. V. Mosby.

Beare, P., Myers, J. (1990). *Principles and practice of adult health nursing.* St. Louis: Mosby–Year Book.

Bennett, J., Brachman, P. (1986). *Hospital infections* (2nd ed). Boston: Little, Brown & Company.

Buczko, G. B., McKay, W. P. S. (1987). Electrical safety in the operating room. *Canadian Journal of Anesthesia* 34:315–322.

Carmody, S., Hickey, P., Bookbinder, M. (1991, July). Perioperative needs of families: Results of a survey. *AORN Journal* 54:561–567.

Centers for Disease Control. (1987, August). Recommendations for prevention of HIV transmission in health-care settings. *Morbidity and Mortality Weekly Report* 36(25).

Council on Scientific Affairs. (1986, August). Lasers in medicine and surgery. *Journal of American Medical Association* 256:900–907.

Cousins, M., Bridenbaugh, P. (1980). *Neural blockade in clinical anesthesia and management of pain.* Philadelphia: J. B. Lippincott.

Covoni, B., Vassallo, H. (1976). *Local anesthetics: Mechanisms of action and clinical use.* New York: Grune & Stratton.

England, E. (1985). Lasers: Issues, problems, and implications for practice. *Perioperative Nursing Quarterly* 1(2):29–38.

Ethicon wound closure manual (1988). Somerville, NJ: Ethicon, Inc.

Fay, M., Beck, W., Fay, J., et al. (1990, June). Medical waste: The growing issues of management and disposal. *AORN Journal* 51:1493–1508.

Fay, M. F. (1987). Drainage systems: Their role in wound healing. *AORN Journal* 46:442–455.

Filston, H., Izant, R. (1985). *The surgical neonate: Evaluation and care.* East Norwalk, Conn: Appleton-Century-Crofts.

Fitzpatrick, B., Reich, R. (1989, October). Sterilization monitoring in vacuum steam sterilizers. *Healthcare Material Management,* 82–85.

Fogg, D. (1989, October). Criteria for flash sterilization. *AORN Journal* 50:888–892.

Fuller, J. R. (1993). *Surgical technology: Principles and practice* (3rd ed). Philadelphia: W. B. Saunders.

Fuller, J. R. (1986). *Surgical technology: Principles and practice* (2nd ed). Philadelphia: W. B. Saunders.

Gillette, M., Caruso, G. (1989, July). Intraoperative tissue injury: Major causes and preventative measures. *AORN Journal* 50:66–78.

Gordon, M. (1987a). *Manual of Nursing: 1986–1987.* New York: McGraw-Hill.

Gordon, M. (1987b.) *Nursing process: Process and application.* New York: McGraw-Hill.

Gorman, N. (1988). Non-woven material: Manufacturing process for sterilization wraps. *Hospital Material Management Quarterly* 9(3):1–8.

Groah, L. (1983). *Operating room nursing: The perioperative role.* Reston, Va: Reston Publishing Co.

Gruendemann, B. J. (1987). *Positioning plus.* Chatsworth, Calif: Deson Industries.

Guyton, A. C. (1991). *Textbook of medical physiology* (8th ed). Philadelphia: W. B. Saunders.

Haney, P., Raymond, B., Lewis, L. (1990, February). Ethylene oxide: An occupational health hazard for hospital workers. *AORN Journal* 52:480–485.

Ignatavicius, D., Batterden, R. A., Hausman, K. A. (1992). *Pocket companion for medical-surgical nursing.* Philadelphia: W. B. Saunders.

Ignatavicius, D., Bayne, M. V. (1991). *Medical-surgical nursing: A nursing process approach.* Philadelphia: W. B. Saunders.

Johnston, C., et al. (1988, January). Parental presence during anesthesia induction: A research study. *AORN Journal* 47:187–194.

Kim, M., Moritz, D. (eds) (1982). *Classification of nursing diagnosis* (p. 258). New York: McGraw-Hill.

Kalapes, A., Greene, V., Langholz, A., et al. (1987). Effect of long-term storage on sterile status of devices in surgical packs. *Infection Control* 8(7):289–293.

Kneedler, J. A., Dodge, G. H. (eds) (1987). *Perioperative nursing care: The nursing perspective* (2nd ed). Boston: Blackwell Scientific.

Kresl, J. S. (1988). Patient-controlled analgesia: A new system for pain management. *AORN Journal* 48:481–487.

Kropp, K. A. (1987). Urology: Surgical aspects. In J. T. Martin (ed), *Positioning in anesthesia and surgery* (2nd ed) (pp. 241–254). Philadelphia: W. B. Saunders.

Larson, E. (1988). APIC guidelines for infection control practice, guideline for use of topical antimicrobial agents. *American Journal of Infection Control* 16:235–266.

Lineweaver, W., Howard, R., Soucy, D., et al. (1985). Topical antimicrobial toxicity. *Archives of Surgery* 120:267–270.

Loving, T., Allen, R. (1985, March/April). EtO personnel monitoring devices: The state of the art. *Journal of Hospital Supply, Processing and Distribution,* pp. 38–42.

Luckman, J., Sorenson, K. C. (1987). *Medical-surgical nursing: A psychophysiologic approach* (3rd ed). Philadelphia: W. B. Saunders.

Martin, J. T. (ed) (1987). *Positioning in anesthesia and surgery* (2nd ed). Philadelphia: W. B. Saunders.

Martinelli, A. M. (1987). Pain and ethnicity: How people of different cultures experience pain. *AORN Journal* 46:273–281.

Masiak, M. J., Naylor, M. D., Hayman, L. L. (1985). *Fluid and electrolytes throughout the life cycle.* East Norwalk, Conn: Appleton-Century-Crofts.

McAlpine, F. S., Seckel, B. R. (1987). *Complications of positioning: The peripheral nervous system* (2nd ed) (pp. 303–328). Philadelphia: W. B. Saunders.

McIlvaine, W. B., Knox, R. F., Fennessey, P. V., Goldstein, M. (1988). Continuous infusion of bupivacaine via intrapleural catheter for analgesia after thoracotomy in children. *Anesthesiology* 69:261–264.

Meeker, M., Rothrock, J. (1991). *Alexander's care of the patient in surgery* (9th ed). (pp. 33–39). St. Louis: Mosby–Year Book.

Melonakos, K. (1990). *Pocket reference for nurses.* Philadelphia: W. B. Saunders.

Miller, K. M. (1987). Deep breathing relaxation: A pain management technique. *AORN Journal* 45:484–488.

Miller, R. D. (1986). *Anesthesia* (2nd ed). New York: Churchill Livingstone.

Mock, E. (1991, March). Electrosurgical unit safety: The role of the perioperative nurse. *AORN Journal* 53:744–752.

Moddeman, G. (1991, May). The elderly surgical patient: A high risk for hypothermia. *AORN Journal* 53:1270–1272.

Moss, R. (1986, May). Overcoming fear: A review of research on patient, family instruction. *AORN Journal* 43:1107–1114.

Moss, V. (1988, July). Music and the surgical patient: The effect of music on anxiety. *AORN Journal* 48:64–69.

National Institute for Occupational Safety and Health. (1989). Ethylene oxide sterilizers in health care facilities, engineering controls and work practices. *Current Intelligence Bulletin* July:52.

Nora, P. F. (1991). *Operative surgery: Principles and techniques* (3rd ed). Philadelphia: W. B. Saunders.

Nyamathi, A., Kashiwabara, A. (1988, January). Preoperative anxiety: Its affect on cognitive thinking. *AORN Journal* 47:164–170.

Phippen, M. L., Well, M. A. (1993). *Perioperative nursing practice.* Philadelphia: W. B. Saunders.

Polk, H. S., Stone, H. H., Gardener, B. (eds) (1987). *Basic surgery* (3rd ed). East Norwalk, Conn: Appleton-Century-Crofts.

Prentice, J. A., Martin, J. T. (1987). The Trendelenburg position: Anesthesiologic considerations. In J. T. Martin (ed), *Positioning in anesthesia and surgery* (2nd ed) (pp. 127–145). Philadelphia: W. B. Saunders.

Regis, M. L., Hill, S. B., Schmidt, C. V. (1986). Wolff-Parkinson-White syndrome: Cryosurgical ablation of accessory pathways. *AORN Journal* 44:742–756.

Rodeheaver, G., Bellamy, W., Kody, M., et al. (1982). Bactericidal activity and toxicity of iodine-containing solutions in wounds. *Archives of Surgery* 117:181–185.

Rothrock, J. C. (ed) (1990). *Perioperative nursing care planning.* St. Louis: Mosby–Year Book.

Rothrock, J. C. (ed) (1987). *The RN first assistant: An expanded perioperative nursing role.* Philadelphia: J. B. Lippincott.

Ryan, P. (1987, November/December). Concepts of cleaning technologies and processes. *Journal of Healthcare Material Management,* 20–27.

Smith, B. L. (1987). The traditional supine position. In J. T. Martin (ed), *Positioning in anesthesia and surgery* (2nd ed) (pp. 33–35). Philadelphia: W. B. Saunders.

Smith, R. (1986, July/August). Sterile: The ten parameters of steam sterilization. *Journal of Healthcare Material Management* ••:34–39.

Salvatiarra, O. (1986). Donor-specific transfusions in living-related transplantation. *World Journal of Surgery* 10:361–368.

Santa Rosa Hospital. (1988). *Laboratory policy and procedure book.* San Antonio: Santa Rosa Hospital.

Santa Rosa Hospital. (1989). *Hazardous communication book.* San Antonio: Santa Rosa Hospital.

Spry, C. (1988). *Essentials of perioperative nursing: A self-learning guide.* Rockville, Md: Aspen Publishers.

Starten, E. D., Cullen, M. L. (1986). Collective review: Epidural catheter analgesia for the management of postoperative pain. *Surgery, Gynecology and Obstetrics* 162:389–404.

Thomas, A. N. (1987). The lateral decubitus position: Surgical aspects. In J. T. Martin (ed), *Positioning in anesthesia and surgery* (2nd ed) (pp. 147–154). Philadelphia: W. B. Saunders.

Thomas, C. L. (ed) (1976). *Taber's cyclopedic medical dictionary.* Philadelphia: F. A. Davis.

Toth, S. (1983). *Patient teaching: A nursing process approach instructor's guide.* Westport, Conn: J. B. Lippincott.

Ulrich, S. P., Canale, S. W., Wendell, S. A. (1986). *Nursing care planning guides: A nursing diagnosis approach.* Philadelphia: W. B. Saunders.

Vidor, K. (1990, September). Anxiety related to impending surgery. *Today's OR Nurse* 12(9):36.

Viljanto, J. (1980). Disinfection of surgical wounds without inhibition of normal wound healing. *Archives of Surgery* 115:253–256.

Wolff, L., Weitzel, M. H., Zornow, R. A., Zsohar, H. (1983). *Fundamentals of nursing* (7th ed). Philadelphia: J. B. Lippincott.

Yura, H., Walsh, M. (1983). *The nursing process: Assessing, planning, implementing, evaluation* (4th ed). East Norwalk, Conn: Appleton-Century-Crofts.

Index

Note: Page numbers in *italics* refer to illustrations; page numbers followed by t refer to tables.

ISBN 0-7216-3412-5

90016

9 780721 634128